Complications of Pregnancy

Edited by Hassan Abduljabbar

Published in London, United Kingdom

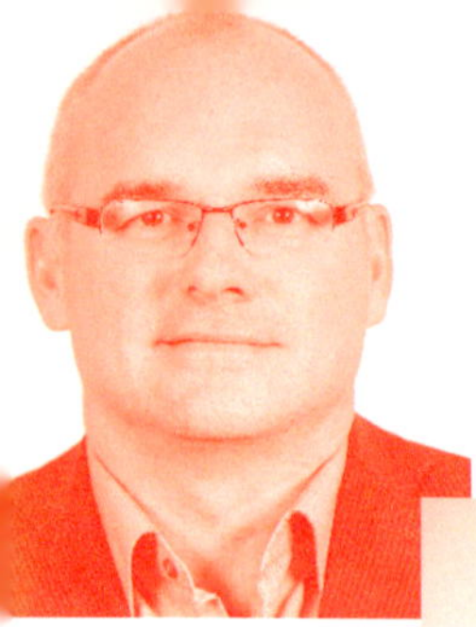
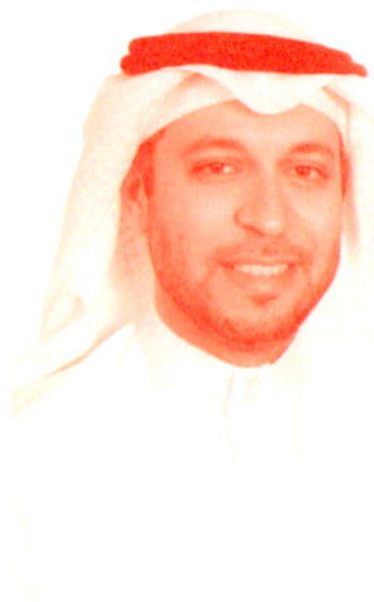
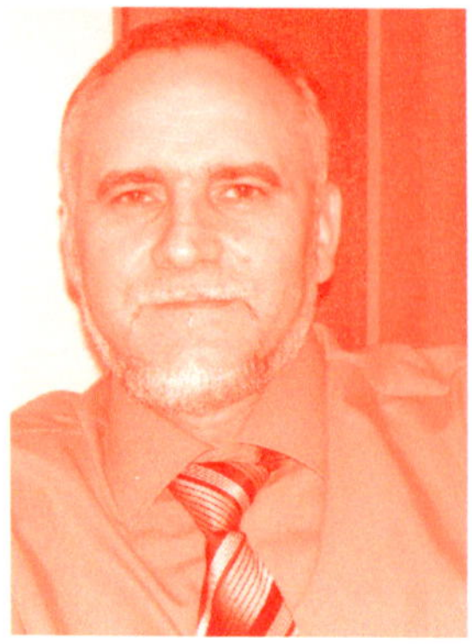
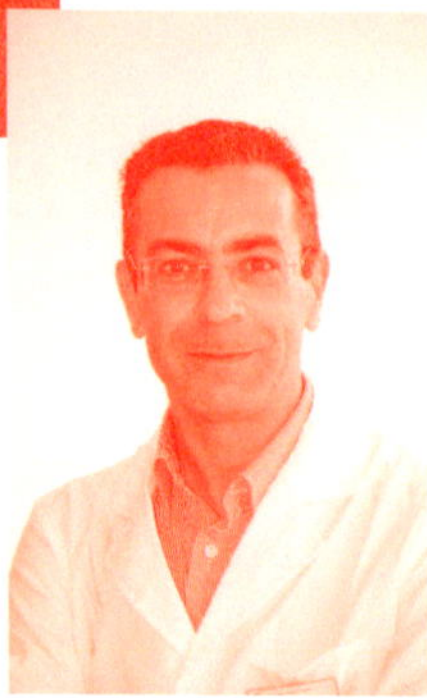
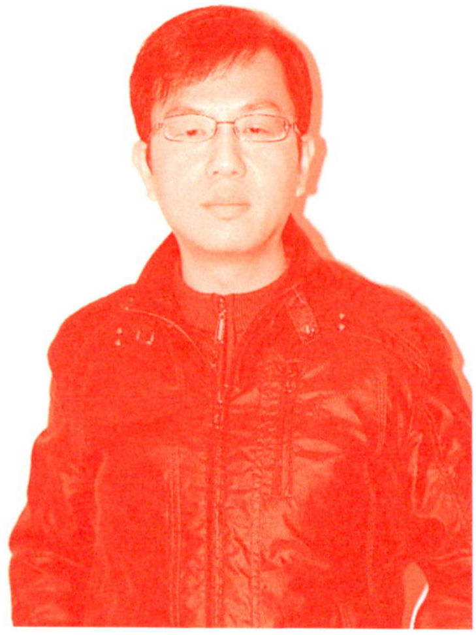
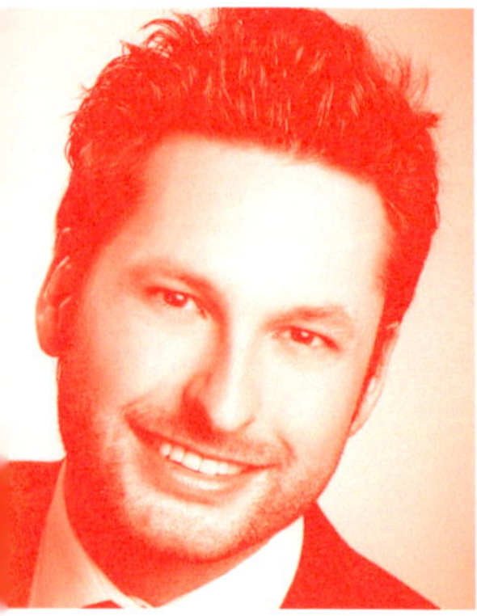
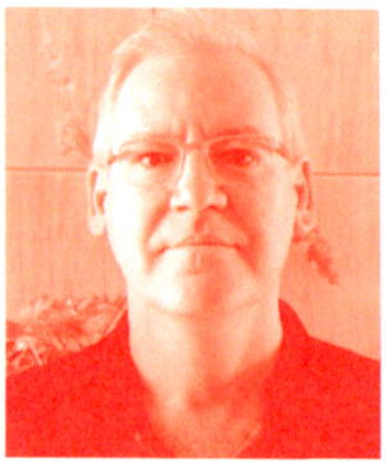

IntechOpen

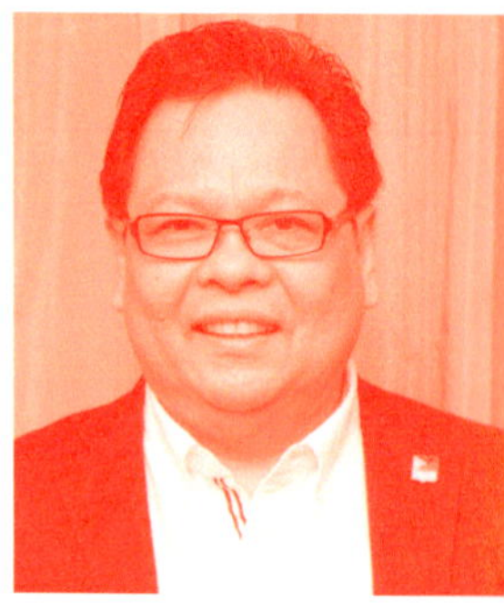
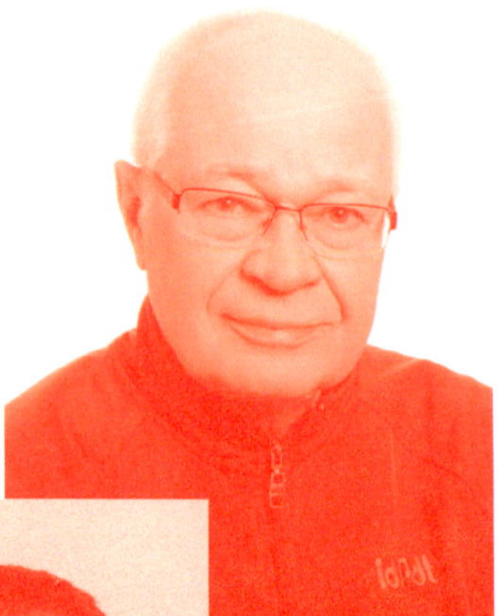
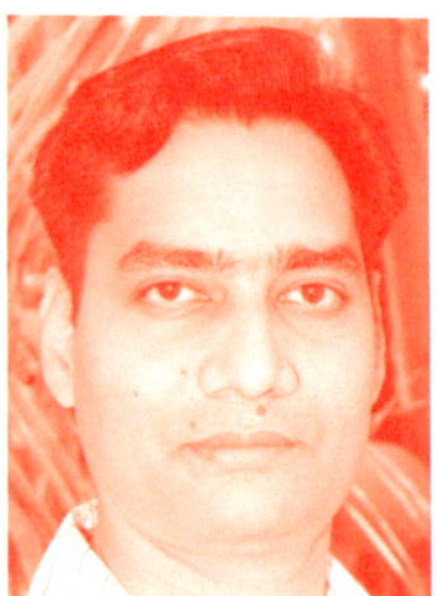
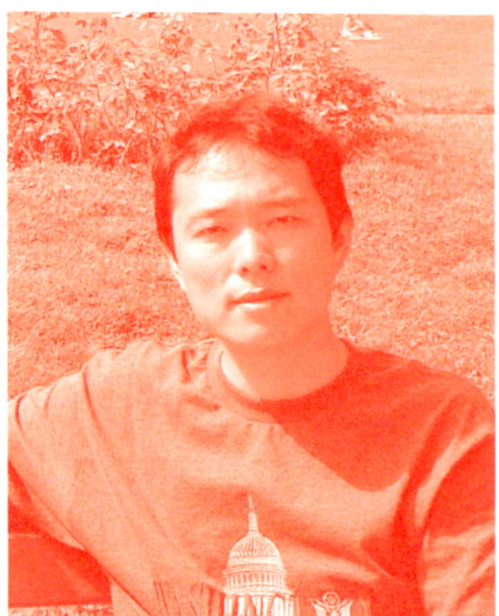
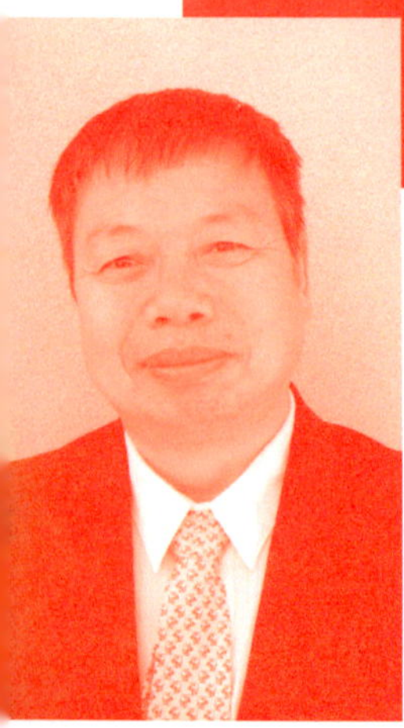
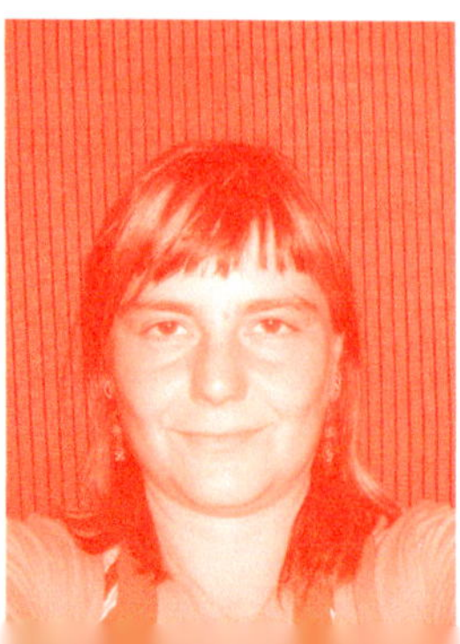

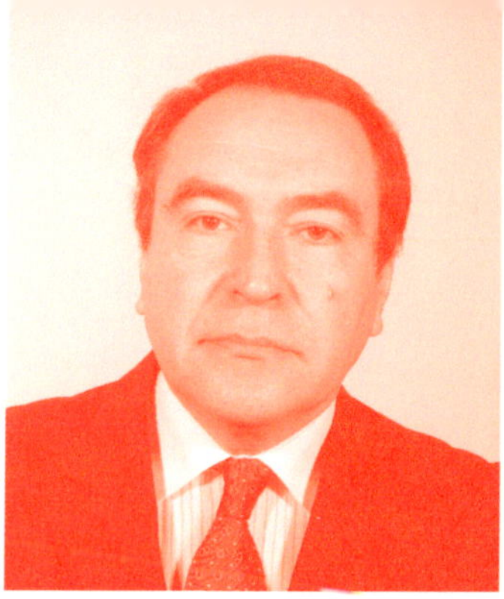
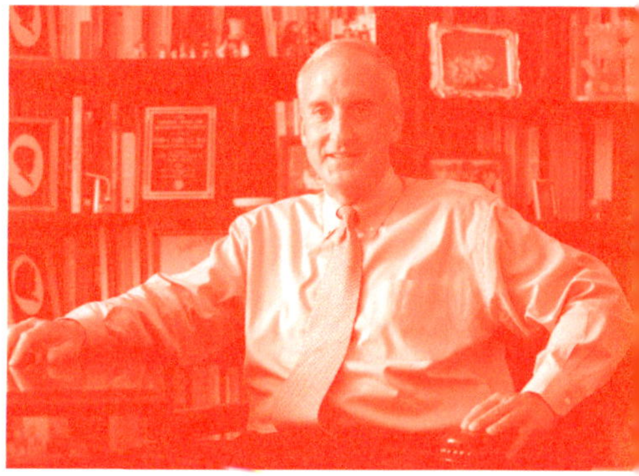
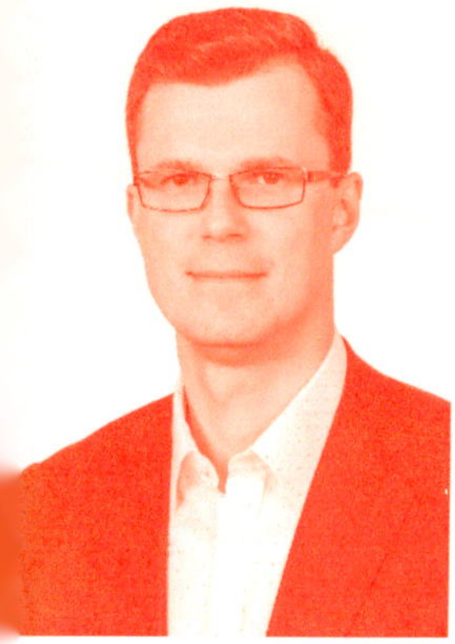
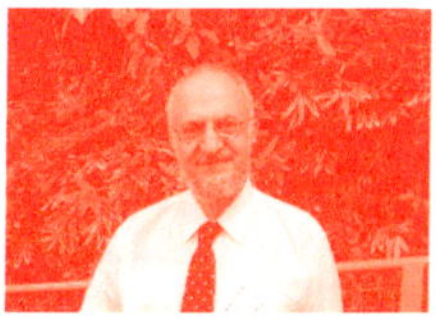
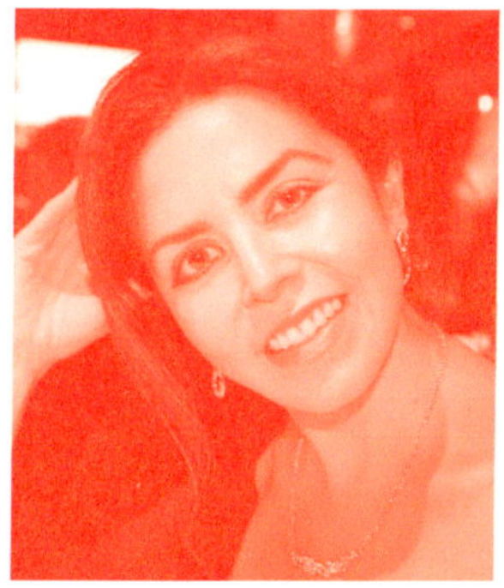

Supporting open minds since 2005

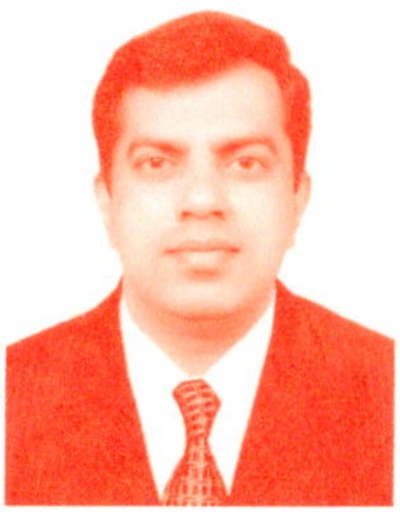
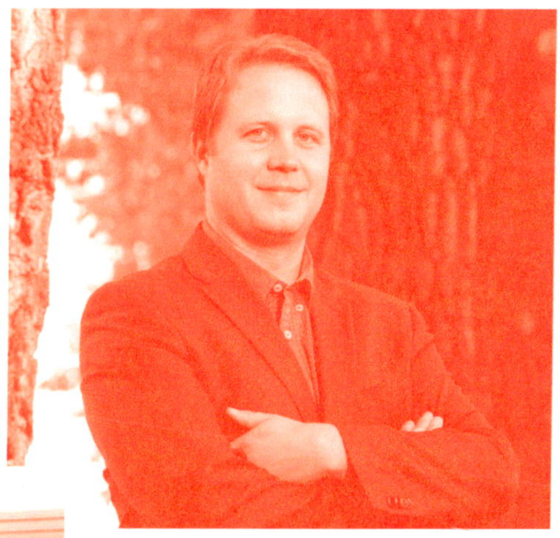
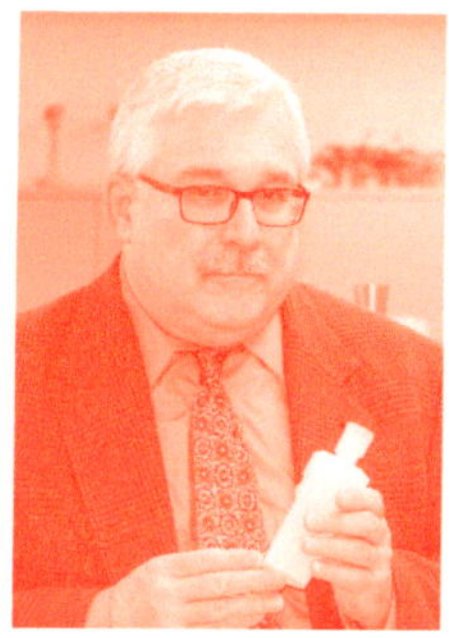
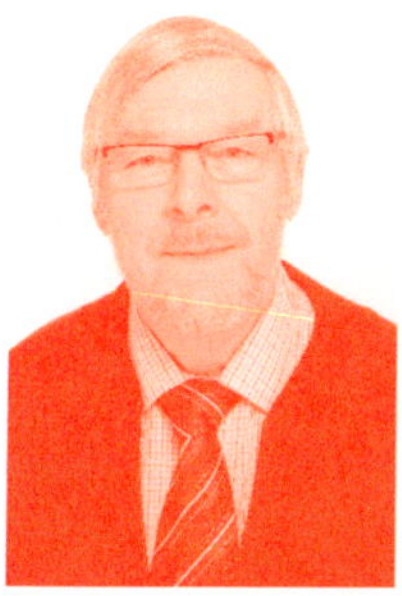
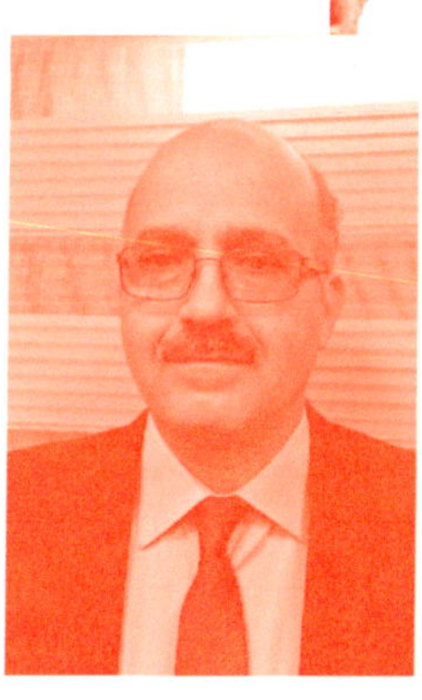
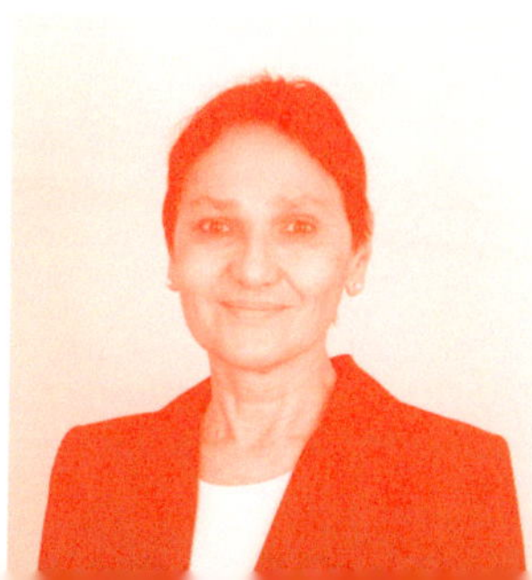
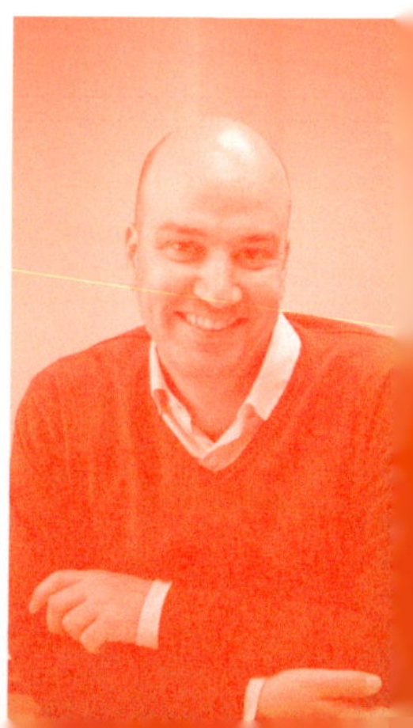

Complications of Pregnancy
http://dx.doi.org/10.5772/intechopen.73930
Edited by Hassan Abduljabbar

Contributors
Alexander Juusela, Rosemary Ogu, John Ojule, Meenakshi Singh, Jyoti Rajak, Sunil Rajadhyaksha, Shalaka Kadam, Renuka Sekar, Sonia Jurado, Kaelly Saraiva, Cauane Marceliano, Vanessa Souza, Izabela Vieira, Hong Soo Wong, Anh Hoang Nguyen

First published in London, United Kingdom, 2019 by IntechOpen
IntechOpen is the global imprint of INTECHOPEN LIMITED, registered in England and Wales, registration number: 11086078, The Shard, 25th floor, 32 London Bridge Street
London, SE19SG – United Kingdom
Printed in Croatia

British Library Cataloguing-in-Publication Data
A catalogue record for this book is available from the British Library

Additional hard copies can be obtained from orders@intechopen.com

Complications of Pregnancy
Edited by Hassan Abduljabbar
p. cm.
Print ISBN 978-1-83880-488-6
Online ISBN 978-1-83880-489-3
eBook (PDF) ISBN 978-1-83880-489-3

For EU product safety concerns:
IN TECH d.o.o., Prolaz Marije Krucifikse Kozulić 3, 51000 Rijeka, Croatia, info@intechopen.com or visit our website at intechopen.com.

Meet the editor

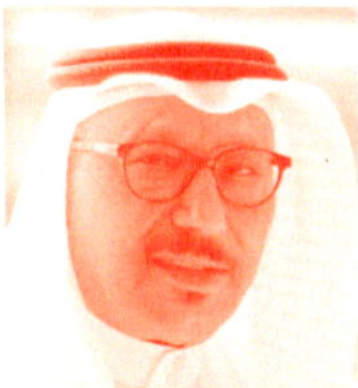

Hassan S. Abduljabbar, MD, FRCSC, American Board Diplomat, is a professor of the Medical College, King Abdulaziz University, and the president of the Saudi Society of Obstetrics and Gynecology. He is a graduate of King Abdulaziz University, June 1980, and College of Medicine & Allied Health Sciences, Jeddah, Saudi Arabia, with an MD (overall grade: excellent secondary honor). He obtained his Royal College of Physicians and Surgeons of Canada degree FRCS (C) in November 1986 after four years of training at the University of Western Ontario. Then, in December 1988, he obtained American Board of Obstetrics and Gynecology certification.
He was the chairman of the Department of Obstetrics and Gynecology and is now the president of the Saudi Society of Obstetrics and Gynecology. He is a referee of many international scientific medical journals and an examiner of Master degrees and PhD degrees as well as in the Saudi and Arab Examination Board. He writes weekly scientific subjects in local newspapers (*Al Bilad*).
His publications in local and international journals exceed 50 articles. He is the editor of three books, *Steroid Basics* (Open Access Books—IntechOpen), *Steroid Clinical* (Open Access Books—IntechOpen), and *Obstetrics* (Open Access Books—IntechOpen), and a chapter in the book *Placenta* (Open Access Books—IntechOpen). He is also the author of 100 MCQ books for medical students. He has four books in the Arabic language.

Contents

Preface

As editor, I would like to introduce this important book *Complications of Pregnancy*, which is an important subject in our specialty. However, as the subject becomes more subspecialized, the general research becomes ever-more limited.

Selection of the topics was done by authors from different countries interested in publishing their research projects. Seven authors have dedicated their input in the form of chapters with different subjects.

The book will be an education for any healthcare provider regarding the research carried out at several universities concerning the complications of pregnancy. It is the result of many facilitating, researching, and teaching group communications.

It is important to teach healthcare providers skills that are based on research from the field of obstetrics and its complications and ensure that those skills are based on current research.

Obstetrics is a branch of medicine that deals with the medical and surgical care of women during pregnancy and delivery and in the postpartum period [1, 2]. The book deals with complications during pregnancy in the following areas:

1. Basic knowledge

Placental abnormalities and their complications during pregnancy [3].

2. Clinical application

a. How early pregnancy loss and miscarriage can affect maternal health [4].

b. Fetal foot length and its effect on diagnosis and complications [5].

c. Nutrition and maternal heath [6].

d. Fetal hydrops fetalis [7].

3. Maternal morbidity and mortality

a. Maternal and fetal complications due to decreased nitric oxide synthesis during gestation [8].

b. Human leukocyte antigen in alloimmunization during pregnancy [9].

4. Postpartum care

a. Immediately after delivery for up to six to eight weeks, the body goes through a number of changes. Healthcare providers should frequently assess blood pressure, heart rate, and amount of bleeding.

b. Complications such as infection of an episiotomy should be avoided, and wound care and the amount of bleeding need to be monitored. Expect the size of the uterus to shrink and become firmer below the umbilicus. Give advice on breastfeeding as soon as possible, which will help to contract the uterus. Observe for infections (bad smells, etc.) [10].

Hassan Abduljabbar
King Abdul Aziz University,
Saudi Arabia

References

[1] Yakushina TI, Kotov SV, Yakushin MA. Analysis of the course of pregnancy, delivery and postpartum period in women with multiple sclerosis. Almanac of Clinical Medicine Al'm klin med. 2016;(39):82-89

[2] Magowan B. Woman-centered care in pregnancy and childbirth. The Obstetrician & Gynaecologist. 2010;**12**(4):292

[3] Anon. Maternal factors, complications associated with morbidly adherent placenta. Journal of Surgery Pakistan. 2017;**22**(3)

[4] Woods-Giscombé CL, Lobel M, Crandell JL. The impact of miscarriage and parity on patterns of maternal distress in pregnancy. Research in Nursing & Health. 2010;**33**(4):316-328

[5] Gameraddin M et al. Accuracy of fetal foot length measurement in estimation of gestational age and fetal weight in the third trimester of pregnancy. Journal of Health Research and Reviews. 2018;**5**(3):142

[6] Lowensohn RI, Stadler DD, Naze C. Current concepts of maternal nutrition. Obstetrical & Gynecological Survey. 2016;**71**(7):413-426

[7] Bellini C, Hennekam RC. Non-immune hydrops fetalis: A short review of etiology and pathophysiology. American Journal of Medical Genetics Part A. 2012;**158A**(3):597-605

[8] Reiher VS et al. Human platelet antigen antibody induction in uncomplicated pregnancy is associated with HLA sensitization. Transfusion. 2017;**57**(5):1272-1279

[9] Bahrami N, Karimian Z, Bahrami S. Comparing the postpartum quality of life between six to eight weeks and twelve to fourteen weeks after delivery in Iran. Iranian Red Crescent Medical Journal. May 2014;**16**(7)

[10] Stuebe AM. Postpartum care—includes breastfeeding, contraception, postpartum endometritis, and postpartum wound infection. Obstetric Evidence Based Guidelines Series in Maternal-Fetal Medicine. 2012:242-253

Section 1

Basic knowledge

Chapter 1

Placental Abnormalities

Alexander L. Juusela

Abstract

A detailed discussion of normal placental development and physiology is beyond the scope of this chapter and is discussed in other chapters. Instead, this chapter will focus on an overview of congenital placental abnormalities and the obstetrical complications that can arise. The goal of this chapter is to delineate the real-world implications of placental abnormalities and provide the reader with a basis for understanding the other chapters that will delve into microbiology, genomics, immunohistochemistry, and biochemistry of the placenta. The focus of this chapter will be on the developmental anomalies and this chapter will not discuss acquired anomalies (e.g., chorioamnionitis, amnion nodosum, metastatic tumors, and umbilical cord true knots). As the intention of this chapter is to focus on the etiopathogenesis of abnormal placentation, it is not intended to instruct the medical management of the described conditions, and therefore the discussions of management will be brief. The information provided is intended for general knowledge only and is not intended for use in diagnosing or treating a health problem or disease without consultation with a qualified healthcare provider. This chapter is not a substitute for professional medical advice, or treatment for specific medical conditions.

Keywords: abnormal placentation, intrinsic placental abnormalities, implantation abnormalities, placental perfusion, placenta accreta, placenta previa, ectopic pregnancy, abruption, hematoma, vasa previa, circumvallate placenta, chorioangioma, amniotic band sequence, placenta membranacea, battledore placenta, single umbilical artery, velamentous umbilical cord, preterm labor, intrauterine growth retardation, intrauterine fetal demise, pregnancy complications, high-risk pregnancy, maternal-fetal medicine, embryology, fetal development, fetal intervention, obstetrical emergency, fetal surgery

1. Introduction

The placenta is a fascinating organ, unique in that it is critical for human development, yet becomes dispensable once extra-uterine life has begun. During embryogenesis, the placenta functions as the maternal-fetal interface and performs the roles of the lungs, liver, and kidneys for the growing gestation, as well as providing nutrition. Placental development is intriguing in the balancing act performed when invading the maternal endometrium to permit growth of the blastocyst, however, unlike neoplasms, its invasion and growth has set end points, beyond which pathologic states can develop **Pictures 1–6**.

The term *placentation* is defined as the formation or arrangement of the placenta in the body of a woman or female animal. As discussed later in this chapter under the ectopic implantation discussion, the definition of placentation will be extended beyond implantation only in the uterus to "the body".

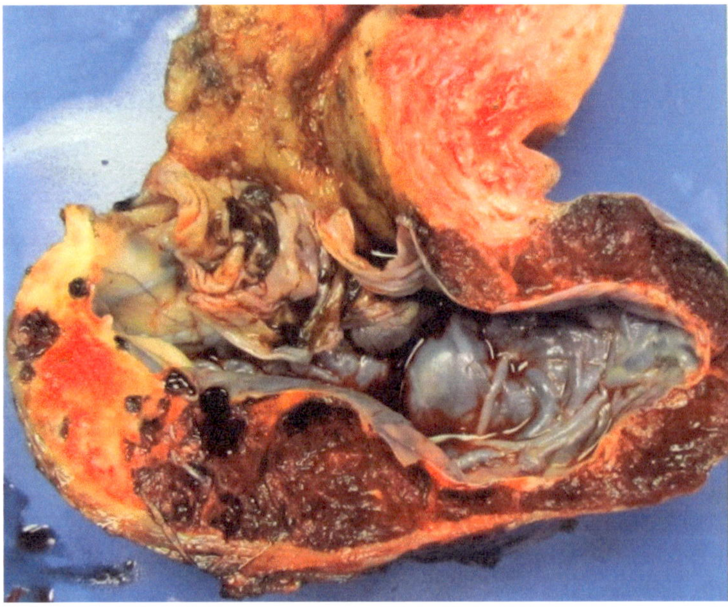

Picture 1.
Placenta previa with placenta accreta.

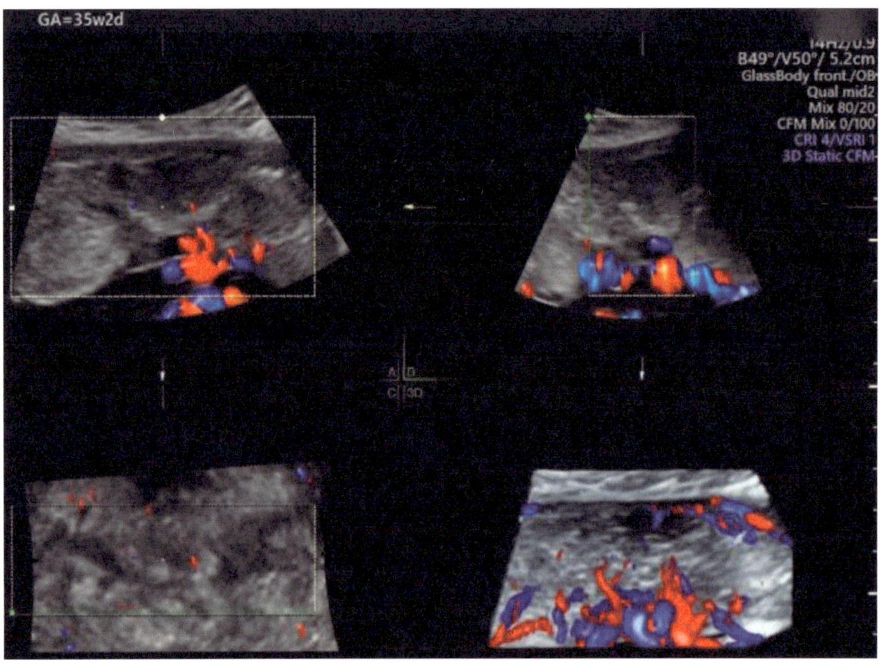

Picture 2.
Increased endometrial invasion by placental vasculature suspicious for placenta accreta.

Over the last couple centuries, scientific investigation has allowed us to understand the embryology, anatomy, and physiology of normal and abnormal placentation on both an organ system and a molecular level. We have established and continue expanding our understanding of how placental abnormalities and malfunctions contribute to the development of maternal, fetal, and neonatal disease, with current investigations examining the correlations between in utero conditions on future disease development during childhood and adulthood. Placental organogenesis, development, function, and malfunction remain fields of vast potential research

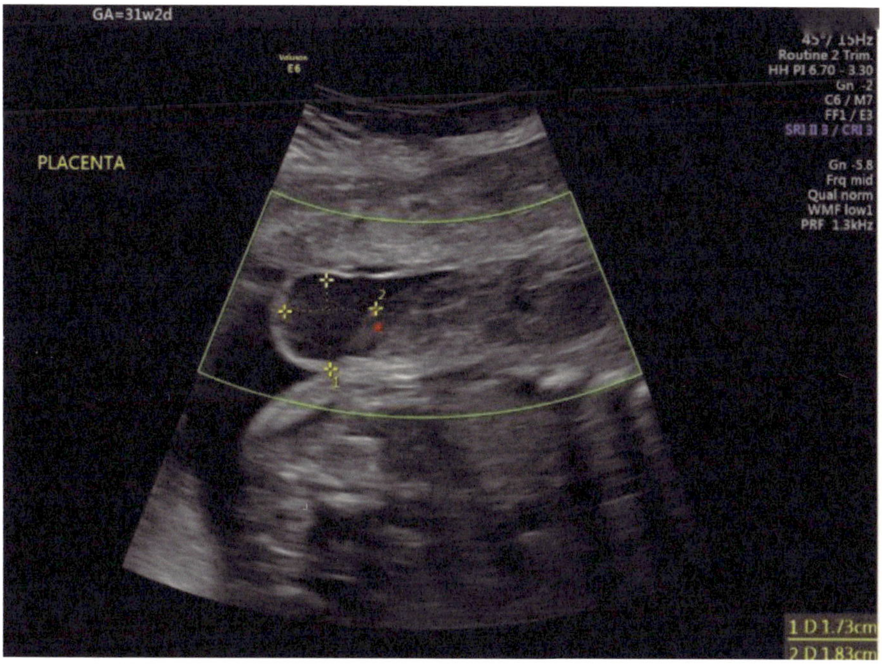

Picture 3.
Placental separation.

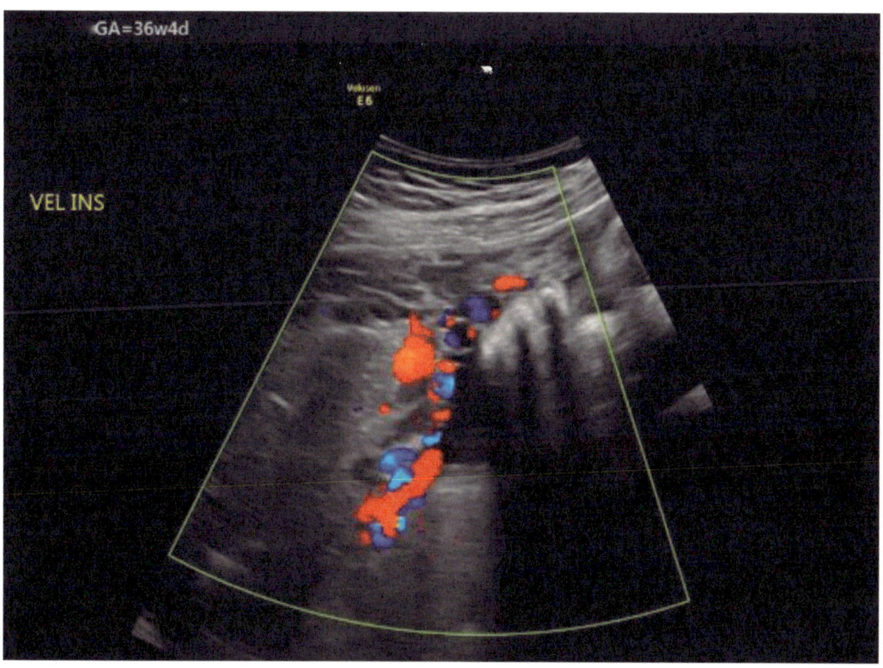

Picture 4.
Velamentous cord insertion.

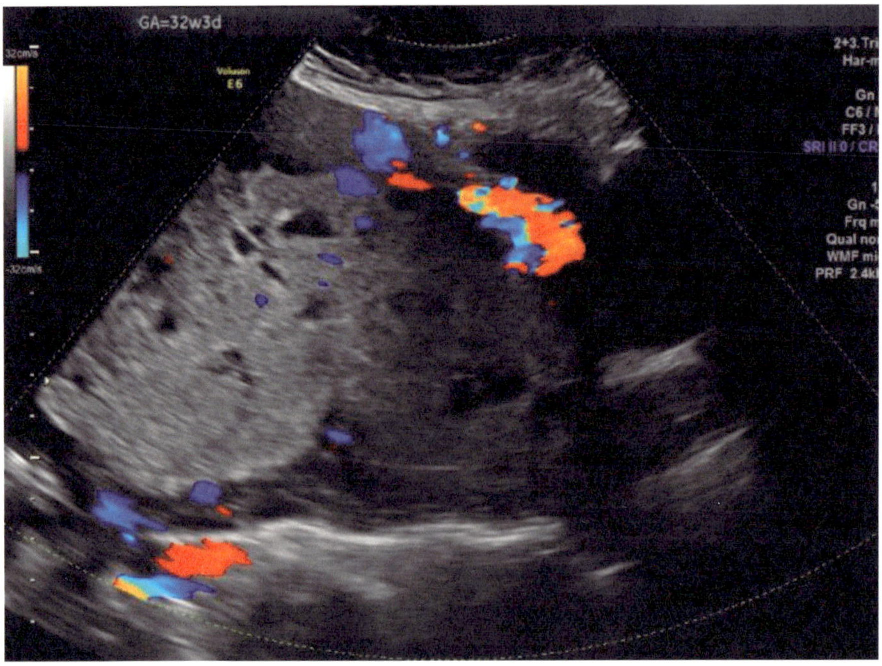

Picture 5.
Placenta previa with placenta percreta invading the bladder.

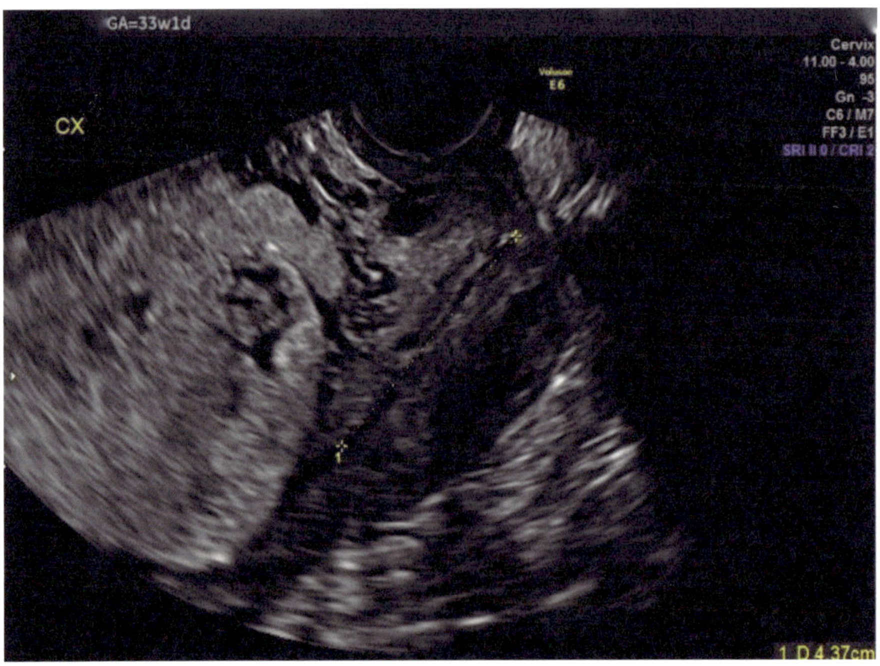

Picture 6.
Placenta previa with measured Cervical Canal.

that are covered in depth in other chapters in this book. The goal of this chapter is to delineate the real-world implications of placental abnormalities and provide the reader with a basis for understanding the other chapters that delve into microbiology, genomics, immunohistochemistry, and biochemistry of the placenta **Table 1**.

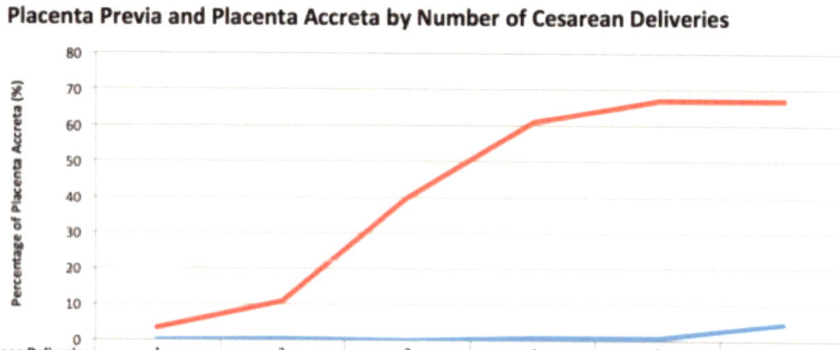

Number of Cesarean Deliveries	1	2	3	4	5	≥6
No Placenta Previa n (%)	0.03	0.2	0.1	0.8	0.8	4.7
Placenta Previa n (%)	3.3	11	40	61	67	67

Table 1.
Placenta previa and placenta accreta by number of cesarean deliveries.

2. Part 1: intrinsic placental abnormalities

A. *Amniotic band syndrome (sequence)*—This congenital structural defect can lead to both minor and major malformations via entanglement of fetal structures in constricting rings. The malformations formed depend on the structure(s) entrapped in the band(s), and can range from minor constriction mediated limb abnormalities, amputation of extremities, complex body wall defects, craniofacial defects, and even gross defects non-compatible with life [1, 2]. The presumed etiopathogenesis leading to the clinical presentation of ABS is that mesodermal bands from the chorionic side of the amnion separate during early gestation and become attached to or entrap the embryo or germ disc [2–5]. Then, as the fetus grows, either via tethering bands or mechanical constriction, malformations develop. There is variance in the definition and debate regarding the associated sequences, complexes, and syndromes. When an abnormal band is noted on prenatal ultrasound, the differential diagnosis must include uterine synechiae, a residual gestational sac, and uterine septa. Once these differential diagnoses are ruled out, further investigation must be taken to identify other fetal or placental abnormalities. To date, there are no known biochemical markers or genes to definitively diagnose the syndrome, however, there is an association with chromosomal abnormalities, and therefore the work-up often includes amniocentesis for karyotype as well as single nucleotide polymorphism (SNP) microarray [6–12]. As the presentation and complications are diverse, management depends on individual cases and ranges from expectant management with intervention in the neonatal/pediatric period, to fetoscopic band transection (fetal surgery), and even termination of pregnancy. The wide range of potential malformations has led to the varied terminology frequently found in the literature, which includes but is not limited to: amniotic band syndrome, amniotic band sequence, amniotic deformity, adhesion mutilation (ADAM) sequence, amniotic band disruption complex, limb body wall complex, body wall complex with limb defects [3–5, 11, 13–18]. The confusion upon review of literature regarding the subject is immediately evident when reviewing the nomenclature. Further investigation is needed to determine if the ABS is a spectrum of one pathologic process or rather a collection of differing pathologic processes which result in similar outcomes.

B. *Bipartite placenta (placenta duplex)*—condition in which the placenta develops into two nearly symmetrical lobes with the umbilical cord insertion inserting between the two lobes. The insertion can either connect with a chorionic bridge or into the membranes (see *velamentous insertion*). A rare condition, placentas with more than two equivalently sized lobes are termed *multilobate*. When a placenta is comprised of two or more unequally sized lobes, the smaller lobe(s) (or *succinturiate lobe*) can develop in the membranes, distal to the primary larger lobe, with connecting vessels running through the membranes in a similar fashion to *velamentous insertion*. The second lobe can sometimes be located quite distant from the main lobe. Placentas with succinturiate lobes are not correlated with adverse fetal effects; it is at the time of labor and delivery that they are subject to the complications. If the succinturiate lobe or connecting vessels are covering the internal cervical os, the risk or vessel avulsion, marginal placental separation, and hemorrhage exist—equivalent to vasa previa and placenta previa. As the succinturiate lobe is often implanted in the membranes, it remains at risk for avulsion and becoming retained at the time of placental removal. This can lead to uterine atony, postpartum hemorrhage, and endometritis.

C. *Chorioangioma*—a benign tumor of the placenta, found in approximately 1% of all pregnancies, which develops from abnormal proliferation of primitive chorionic vessels [19]. *Chorioangiomas* are typically small masses without clinical consequences, however, large *chorioangiomas*, typically lesions larger than 4 cm, can cause hydramnios, arteriovenous (AV) shunting, and fetal red blood cell (RBC) sequestration. AV shunting and RBC sequestration can lead to fetal anemia, non-immune hydrops fetalis, fetal cardiomyopathy, intrauterine fetal growth restriction (IUGR), and even fetal demise [19–22]. *Chorioangiomas* are diagnosed via ultrasonography as well circumscribed solid or complex masses located on the fetal side of the placenta with turbulent hypervascular flow on Doppler-flow imaging. Management depends on the size of the mass, evidence of hydramnios, and evidence of fetal compromise, with management ranging from amnioreduction, percutaneous intrauterine transfusion, and embolization or laser coagulation of feeding vessels [20–22].

D. *Circummarginate placenta*—a rare embryologic abnormality in which hemorrhage and fibrin deposition separate the placenta and amniochorion. This condition is more common in multigravidas and has no known clinical significance. In comparison to circumvallate placenta, there is no firm ridge at the edge of the placenta and the margin is thin and flat. It typically is an incidental finding during prenatal ultrasound.

E. *Circumvallate placentation*—a rare embryologic abnormality in which the chorionic plate is unusually smaller than the basal plate, causing the amniotic membranes to insert medial to the placental edge. On examination, there is a characteristic white ring around the surface of the placental disk that is comprised of a double layer of amnion and chorion with fibrin and necrotic villi. It is predisposed to abnormal separation and commonly presents with 2nd trimester vaginal bleeding, being diagnosed via ultrasound or after delivery [23]. Pregnancy complications are common and include oligohydramnios, small for gestational age (SGA) neonates, abruption, and intrauterine fetal demise (IUFD) [24–26]. Management depends on the individual cases and subsequent maternal and/or fetal complications.

F. *Four-vessel umbilical cord*—During embryogenesis the umbilicus develops initially with two arteries and two veins. During the 1st trimester one umbilical vein atrophies and the normal human placenta develops with one large umbilical vein and two smaller umbilical arteries. Four-vessel umbilical cords are rare phenomena in which both umbilical veins and both arteries remain. This condition is associated with congenital anomalies, and when found should prompt further investigation; however, when it is an isolated finding the clinical prognosis is improved [27–29].

G. *Marginal (battledore) umbilical cord insertion* This condition is called battledore placentation secondary to the shape of the placenta and cord. In this condition, the cord inserts at the edge of the placenta and gives it the appearance of the racquet used in the precursor game to badminton. Marginal umbilical cord insertions are present in approximately 6.3% of singleton gestations and 10.9% in twin gestations, especially in monochorionic twin gestations [30]. This condition rarely causes complications in singleton gestations prior to the 3rd stage of labor, during which, the marginal cord insertion can be avulsed during placental delivery [31]. In monochorionic twin gestations, a marginal cord insertion may lead to unequal sharing of the placental mass and therefore lead to discordant fetal weight [32].

H. *Placenta membranacea*—in this rare condition, the chorionic sac is nearly or completely covered by placental villi. The placenta is thin, yet deeply implanted in the endometrium, which places it at risk for forming placenta accreta and previa, with the subsequent sequellae of the aforementioned conditions. Aside from the risks associated with placenta previa and accreta, placenta membranacea is also at risk for recurrent antepartum bleeding, intra-uterine growth retardation (IUGR), miscarriage, preterm labor, intrauterine fetal demise (IUFD), retained placenta after delivery, and postpartum hemorrhage [33–35].

I. *Single umbilical artery* (SUA)—SUA is an umbilical cord anomaly in which only one umbilical artery develops, and is the most common congenital umbilical cord anomaly. There are currently three proposed mechanisms of action leading to SUA. The first is primary agenesis of one of the umbilical arteries. The second is secondary atresia or atrophy of one artery in a normal three-vessel umbilical cord. The third is persistence of the embryologic single allantoic artery of the body stalk. When a SUA is identified on fetal ultrasonography, further work-up (detailed fetal ultrasonography, fetal echocardiography, and amniocentesis for karyotype) are warranted, as there is an associated high incidence of major chromosomal and congenital anomalies, as well as abnormalities of the renal and cardiac structures [36–41]. SUA is associated with intrauterine growth retardation (IUGR), preterm labor (PTL), small-for-gestational-dates (SGA) neonates, and the aforementioned structural anomalies. Twin gestations are affected in approximately 4–11%, without a difference in incidence between monochorionic and dichorionic twins [42]. When isolated SUA (iSUA) is identified, the fetus usually has normal chromosomes, and routine neonatal examination and care is indicated [43].

J. *Succinturiate placental lobe(s)*—see *Bipartite placenta* for discussion.

K. *Vasa previa*—an uncommon condition occurring in an estimated 0.60 per 1000 pregnancies, in which, like to *velamentous umbilical cord*, the vessels pass within the membranes and cross over the internal cervical os [44]. In fact, *vasa previa* is often identified in conjunction with *placenta previa*, a *velamentous cord, succinturiate lobes*, and in the setting of in vitro fertilization (IVF). These vessels are also at risk of compression when fetal parts become engaged with the cervix. Equivalent to velamentous insertion, vasa previa is at risk of vessel avulsion during membrane rupture and cervical dilation. Upon vessel avulsion, the fetus can precipitously exsanguinate, therefore, prenatal diagnosis is paramount in preventing potentially catastrophic peripartum complications [45]. The diagnostic modality of choice is transvaginal ultrasound with Doppler flow [46–48]. When diagnosed in the antepartum period, the preferred method of birth is planned cesarean delivery prior to the onset of labor or rupture of membranes.

L. *Velamentous insertion of the umbilical cord*—a potentially catastrophic umbilical cord anomaly in which the umbilical vessels separate in the membranes before the cord reaches the chorionic plate. The vessels are not covered by Wharton's jelly and can therefore be easily compressed, lacerate, and rupture, leading to fetal hemorrhage [46]. The vessels are at greatest risk with rupturing of membranes as the vessels can tear. A common presenting sign is increased vaginal bleeding at the time of spontaneous rupture of membranes (SROM) or artificial rupture of membranes (AROM) [49]. Pregnancies complicated by velamentous insertion of the umbilical cord are associated with increased risk of PPROM, preterm labor, abruption, peripartum non-reassuring fetal heart tracing (NRFHT), cord avulsion requiring manual removal of the placenta, cesarean delivery, and fetal/neonatal death [31, 46, 49, 50]. When diagnosed in the antepartum period, management depends on whether or not the velamentous cord insertion is associated with vasa previa. When it is associated with vasa previa, the preferred method of birth is planned cesarean delivery prior to the onset of labor or rupture of membranes. In the absence of vasa previa, there is currently no evidence that cesarean delivery or induction of labor improve outcomes. As the vessels lack the Wharton's Jelly found in normal umbilical cords, the vessels are prone to compression and avulsion, therefore laboring patients should have continuous fetal heart rate monitoring to allow prompt diagnosis of fetal distress. Additionally, there is an increased risk of cord avulsion when traction is applied to the umbilical cord in the third stage of labor.

3. Part 2: implantation abnormalities

A. Abnormal implantation

a. *Ectopic implantation* (ectopic pregnancy) occurs when the blastocyst implants in a site other than the uterine endometrium and is estimated at between 0.5 and 1.5% of all 1st trimester pregnancies in the United States [51, 52]. Ectopic implantation is most common in the fallopian tube (approximately 96% of ectopic pregnancies) [53], but it can occur in the uterine cornua, ovary, cervix, and even parasitically implanting into the intraabdominal organs and vessels [54–58]. Unlike the uterus, structures like the fallopian tube, cervix, cesarean scar, and ovary cannot accommodate a growing fetus, are prone to acute rupture, and the resulting hemorrhage can be life threatening. The current era in medicine, with diagnostic modalities such as ultrasound and Beta-HCG hormone blood and urine level testing, diagnosing ectopic pregnancy rapidly has led to decreased morbidity and mortality. In the United States, the mortality rate from ectopic pregnancy has decreased since the 1980s, with ectopic pregnancy comprising 3% of all cause pregnancy-related deaths in a 2017 study [59, 60]. Risk factors for ectopic pregnancy include history of sexually transmitted or other pelvic infection (such as chlamydia, gonorrhea, pelvic inflammatory disease and tubo-ovarian abscess), prior ectopic pregnancy, tubal surgery, tobacco smoking, pelvic adhesions (e.g., secondary to endometriosis, salpingitis, pelvic abscess, appendicitis), assisted reproductive technology, congenital fallopian tube abnormalities, diethylstilbestrol exposure, and Salpingitis isthmica nodosa [61–63]. Patient presentation and outcomes depend on the pregnancy location and range from pregnancy failure with reabsorption, to spontaneous abortion, to continued growth leading to surrounding structure rupture and hemorrhage. Management depends on a multitude of factors including the site of implantation, size of the gestational sac or fetus, beta-human chorionic gonadotropin (Beta-HCG) hormone level, and the patient's presenting signs and symptoms and range from expectant management, to intragestational or systemic methotrexate (MTX), to surgical intervention.

b. *Placenta previa* is the term when placental implantation is either adjacent to or covering the internal cervical os. The prevalence varies per region, however, has been estimated between approximately 4 and 5.2 per 1000 pregnancies, with the incidence of marginal placenta previas decreasing as gestational age increases (see discussion below for further details) [64, 65]. Further distinction is made between complete coverage of the internal cervical os or *complete placenta previa* versus when the leading edge of the placenta is implanted within less than 2 cm from the internal cervical os or *marginal placenta previa*. The severity of complications varies widely based on the location of the placenta in relation to the cervical os, as well as the degree of placental separation. The location of the placenta over or at the margin of the internal cervical os leads to a predisposition for hemorrhage if cervical dilation occurs as any cervical dilation will expose placental blood vessels, leading to a range from concealed bleeding (i.e., no observed vaginal bleeding) to frank exsanguination. Complications during labor arise from both the placental separation and the structural blockage of fetal expulsion from the uterus by a complete previa. Depending on the placental implantation site, as the uterus grows throughout the gestation, marginal placenta previas, when followed by serial ultrasound examination have a documented tendency to become progressively distanced away from the internal cervical os. However, placenta previa remains at risk of interface separation and subsequent hemorrhage when contractions and/or cervical dilation occur at any time during the pregnancy. The etiopathogenesis of placenta previa remains elucidated, and the two current hypotheses are: 1. Lack of a suitable implantation site in the uterine fundus or corpus. Secondary to uterine trauma from previous surgery (e.g., cesarean deliveries, myomectomies, dilation & curettage) and/or multiple pregnancies, the sites of normal implantation develop areas of suboptimally vascularized uterine decidua, which predispose to implantation of the trophoblast in the lower uterine segments [64]. 2. Large placental surface area, secondary to conditions such as multiple gestations and *placenta membranacea*, increases the probability of the placenta implanting or extending over the internal cervical os. Known major risk factors include: 1. Previous placenta previa, which has a recurrence in 4–8% of future pregnancies [64, 66, 67]. 2. Previous Cesarean deliveries, with a dose–response pattern in the risk of placenta previa, the risk increasing with the number of cesarean deliveries previously performed [68, 69]. 3. Multiple gestations—in a retrospective cohort study that included 67,895 pregnancies, 2.1% of singleton and 2.5% of twin gestations had previa diagnosed. A subgroup analysis demonstrated that dichorionic twin gestations were at an increased risk for ultrasonography-diagnosed previa when compared with monochorionic or single gestations [70]. Minor risk factors include: 1. Increasing maternal age. 2. Increasing parity. 3. Previous non-cesarean delivery surgeries (uterine evacuation, myomectomy, infertility procedures). 4. Drug usage (tobacco smoking and cocaine usage). 5. Non-white race. 6. Male fetus. Management of placenta previa depends on if it is a complete or marginal previa, if there is a suspected concomitant placenta accreta, and then individualized based on multiple factors: the estimated gestational age (EGA), the distance of the placental edge from the internal cervical os, any evidence of abruption, maternal vaginal bleeding, hemodynamic instability, or evidence of fetal distress. Therefore obstetricians must base management on their assessment of individual cases. An actively bleeding placenta previa is a potential obstetrical emergency, and should be handled as if having the potential for rapid hemorrhage and requirement for massive transfusion of blood products and crystalloid. Upon the onset of labor, if both the mother and fetus are stable, and the placenta is at least 2 cm from the internal cervical os, the patient can safely undergo labor.

c. *Placenta accreta spectrum (PAS)*—a collection of conditions of abnormal placentation caused by trophoblastic invasion into the myometrial tissue beyond the normal boundary established by the Nitabuch fibrinoid layer. The PAS includes the diagnoses of *placenta accreta, increta and percreta*, with the definitions differing solely based on the depth of invasion of the placenta into the uterus and even beyond the uterus into adjacent structures and organs. Whereas, in normal placentation, placental villi attach to the decidual basalis, microscopic analysis of PAS has demonstrated partial or complete absence of the decidual layer such that the placental villi attach and/or interdigitate with myometrial fibers [71–75]. Mechanical disruption of the endometrial tissue from cesarean deliveries, myomectomies, uterine ablation, dilation and curettage, or endometritis is the current leading hypothesized etiopathogenesis of PAS [71–79]. Investigation is currently underway to identify other factors such as increased growth expression and angiogenesis that may contribute this pathologic process [75, 76, 80]. Physiologically, separation between placental cotyledons and the uterus occurs at the decidual layer, which functions as a cleavage line. In the absence of a decidual layer, separation between the placental cotyledons and the uterine spiral arteries does not occur, and the uterus continues to perfuse the cotyledons, which, in turn, leads to hemorrhage [77]. The current estimated incidence of PAS is 3.0 per 1000 pregnancies [81]. Secondary to the rise in frequency of operative procedures (specifically cesarean deliveries, with an estimated incidence increasing from 12.5% in 1982 to 32.2% in 2014 [78, 81]), there was a concomitant estimated increase in PAS of 0.8 per 1000 deliveries during the 1980s to the current estimate of 3.0 per 1000 pregnancies [78, 81–86]. Undiagnosed PAS can lead to massive intrapartum and postpartum hemorrhage, consumptive coagulopathy, disseminated intravascular coagulopathy, hypovolemic shock, and maternal mortality [71, 79, 87, 88]. The importance of antepartum placental analysis has been well established, and the individual practitioner must have a high index of suspicion at the time of delivery [89]. US and magnetic resonance imaging (MRI) are the diagnostic modalities most frequently used [90–93]. Identification of placental invasion of the myometrium can be made with US, with a positive predictive value (PPV) of 68%, a negative predictive value (NPV) of 98%, and a sensitivity of 89.5% [90]; with MRI, the sensitivity is 88%, specificity is 100%, PPV is 100%, and NPV is 82% [91]. Establishing a suspected diagnosis of PAS before delivery allows for a scheduled delivery and pre-operative planning with a multidisciplinary team based on the severity of the PAS. This can include consultation with a Maternal-Fetal Medicine specialists, gynecologic-oncologists, general surgeons, urologists, vascular surgeons, anesthesiologists, neonatologists, intensive care specialists, interventional radiologists, blood bank personnel, and nursing staff. There currently is inconclusive evidence for improved outcomes with pre-delivery placement of ureteral stents or internal iliac artery occlusive devices. Management of PAS varies as widely as the degree of abnormal placentation. Case by case management depends on whether or not it was identified before delivery, estimated gestational age (EGA), maternal factors (co-morbidities, previous surgery, status of labor), the size of the morbidly adherent placenta, the hemorrhage encountered, structures invaded by the placenta, adhesions, parity, presence of placenta previa, and other individualized factors. No randomized controlled trials (RCT) exist to guide management; therefore management varies between institutions and practitioners. The definitive treatment for PAS is cesarean-hysterectomy; however, experimental modalities aimed at uterine conservation have included leaving the placenta en situ followed by hypogastric artery ligation, uterine artery embolization, compression sutures, intrauterine balloon tamponade, and adjuvant methotrexate [94]. It should be noted that these experimental methods remain at risk for hemorrhage and delayed hysterectomy. It is the opinion of both the American College of Obstetricians and Gynecologists (Committee Opinion No. 529) as well as this author, that cases should be individualized, but "the recommended management of suspected placenta accreta is planned preterm cesarean hysterectomy with the placenta left in situ." [95] If the practitioner believes that adequate care cannot be administered, then transfer of care to a tertiary care center, specifically a center of excellence for PAS, is recommended.

d. *Cervical ectopic pregnancy* is a rare phenomenon, estimated at <1% of all ectopic pregnancies [57], while *cervical placenta accreta* is an even rarer condition. In contrast to the endometrium, the cervix does not contain a decidual layer; therefore, it is hypothesized that pathogenesis of cervical accretas is attributable to direct damage from cervical instrumentation during in vitro fertilization, intrauterine device placement, dilation and curettage, cesarean delivery, and previous cervical and/or uterine surgery [96, 97]. While diagnosis of a cervical ectopic pregnancy is made via ultrasound, cervical placenta accreta is a pathologic diagnosis made after surgical procedures such as trachelectomy and hysterectomy. Therefore, management is that of a cervical ectopic pregnancy. Ultrasound has allowed for early diagnosis and attempts at preservation of reproductive capacity via intragestational potassium chloride or methotrexate (MTX), local or systemic MTX, and/or uterine and hypogastric artery embolization [57, 96, 97]. However, when conservative measures fail in the acute scenario, the conventional gold standard remains total abdominal hysterectomy (TAH) [98].

B. Abnormal cytotrophoblastic invasion

a. Implantation of the blastocyst into the endometrium occurs between days 6 and 7 after fertilization and is a highly regulated process that occurs in three phases: 1. Apposition, or initial contact of the blastocyst with the endometrium; 2. Adhesion, or adhesion between the blastocyst and decidua, and; 3. Invasion, or continued penetration into and invasion of the decidua by the syncytiotrophoblast and cytotrophoblasts, down to the inner third of the myometrium, followed by union with the uterine vasculature. Studies are currently underway to identify the exact pathways and mechanisms by which the blastocyst, like a neoplasm, invades the decidua, inner third of the myometrium, and stimulates local angiogenesis to promote its own growth [99, 100]. Unlocking this complex process has enormous potential for the fields of oncology and reproductive endocrinology [101]. Investigation into the three phases of implantation have identified numerous growth factors [e.g., vascular endothelial growth factor (VEGF), placental growth factor (PlGF), transforming growth factor-B1 (TGF-B1)], angiogenic factors, adhesion molecules, cytokines, interleukins, receptors, transcription factors, and associated pathways [102–105]. For example, adhesion of the blastocyst to the endometrium depends on hormonally mediated Integrins, one of the four classes of cell receptors termed cellular adhesion molecules (CAMs) [106–108]. The mechanisms of impaired trophoblast migration are also currently being elucidated, and are associated with local placental hypoxia and abnormal placental growth factors, including placental growth factor (PlGF), hypoxia inducible factor (HIF), tyrosine kinase 1 (sFlt1), and reactive oxygen species [109–111]. Defective implantation and placentation clinically leads to recurrent spontaneous abortion, PPROM, IUGR, and preterm labor [112]. Inadequate or absence of secondary invasion of the endovascular trophoblast into the maternal spiral arteries of the myometrial layers during weeks 15 to 22 of gestation is associated with maternal chronic hypertension (CHTN), preeclampsia, and diabetes [112, 113].

4. Part 3: processes affecting placental perfusion

A. Abnormal placental separation

a. The author acknowledges that there are various medical conditions and mechanisms of action (such as trauma and hypertension) that can lead to abnormal placental separation, however, this topic is included in this chapter as current investigation is underway correlating genetics and characteristics of certain placentas to a predisposition for abnormal placental separation. The pathways and cascades that interact to prevent or promote separation and rupture of membranes include cytokines, transcription factors, thrombin, matrix metalloproteinases (MMP), prostaglandins, hormones, collagen, proteoglycans, and fetal fibronectin (FFN) [114–116].

b. *Chorionic hematoma*—a hematoma (collection of blood) between the chorion and the uterine wall. It occurs in an estimated 3.1% of all pregnancies and typically presents with first trimester vaginal bleeding, and is associated with spontaneous abortion when occurring in the first trimester [117]. Sonographically, hematomas appear as hypoechoic crescents with location depending on the type. Chorionic hematomas may mimic a thickened placenta because the hematoma is often isoechoic to the placenta; however, on color Doppler ultrasound there is the absence of internal blood flow. Three types exist:

   i. *Subchorionic hematoma*—the partial detachment of the chorionic membranes from the endometrium due to mass effect by a hematoma. It is the most common form.

   ii. *Subamniotic (preplacental) hematoma*—a rare form of hematoma that is contained within the amnion and chorion.

   iii. *Retroplacental hematomas*—complete or partial detachment of the placenta from the uterine wall with a hematoma confined behind the placenta. When the Large hematomas can decrease trans-placental perfusion and lead to intrauterine growth retardation (IUGR) and oligohydramnios [118].

c. *Placental abruption*—Abnormal placental separation, termed abruption placentae or placental abruption, is defined as the complete or partial separation of a normally implanted placenta from the uterine wall after 20 weeks of gestation, but before delivery of the fetus. This condition affects an estimated 1 in every 100–120 pregnancies and typically presents after 20 week of gestation; however, the gestational age-specific incidences depend on the underlying etiopathogenesis of individual cases [44, 119–121]. Placental abruption is a clinical diagnosis, and even with prompt diagnosis, the maternal and fetal morbidity and mortality can be devastating. The presentation varies from the classic scenario of post-mechanical event (such as trauma) acute-onset painful life-threatening obstetrical hemorrhage with associated fetal distress noted on external fetal monitoring to incidentally identify painless concealed focal retroplacental hematomas with intraplacental anechoic areas to chronic painless vaginal bleeding [122–124]. It should be noted that ultrasound has a low sensitivity for diagnosing abruption, and therefore diagnosis should be based on clinical suspicion. Known risk factors include trauma, hypertensive disorders, preterm premature rupture of membranes (PPROM), subchorionic hematomas, and cocaine [123, 125, 126]. Management is individualized to the degree and severity of individual cases, ranging from emergent cesarean delivery for acute complete abruptions to serial surveillance and expectant management for contained retroplacental hematomas. While management of acute abruptions is part of the standard training for obstetricians, the individualized management of chronic and/or partial abruptions without evidence of fetal compromise or maternal instability is a less defined arena which must take account maternal factors (such as medical co-morbidities, hemoglobin and hematocrit level, blood type, evidence of coagulopathy, Bishop score, and patient reliability for close surveillance) as well as fetal considerations (such as gestational age, viability, fetal presentation, complications, estimated fetal weight, chorionicity, practitioners experience). It is a scenario that often leads to consultation with Maternal-Fetal Medicine specialists for assistance and guidance. The mechanical separation at the maternal-fetal interface can decrease the placental perfusion in a fashion similar to placental infarcts and acute atherosis of the spiral arteries (please see the relevant sections of this chapter) and can lead to fetal acidemia, intrauterine fetal growth restriction (IUGR), small for gestational age (SGA) neonates, chronic abruption-oligohydramnios sequence, and preeclampsia [127–129]. Abruptions with large volume hemorrhage can lead to cardiovascular compromise, disseminated intravascular coagulation (DIC), and both fetal and maternal mortality. Patients with a history of one previous placental abruption are at 3–15% risk of future abruption, and women with a history of two previous abruptions are between 20 and 25% risk of repeat abruption [44, 130–133]. Research focused on preventing placental and maternal interface infarcts is currently active with small randomized controlled trials (RCTs) demonstrating a protective effect with anticoagulants administered in a subcuticular manner [134].

5. Conclusions

The placenta is an indispensable, yet temporary, organ of the developing human that we are rapidly improving our knowledge of via scientific investigation. Clinical correlates of placental abnormalities and malfunction are a common occurrence at prenatal testing centers and on the labor and delivery wards throughout the world. Placental abnormalities can lead to adverse fetal outcomes such as SGA/IUGR, discordant growth in twins, preterm birth, IUFD as well as maternal adverse outcomes such as hemorrhage requiring blood transfusion, surgery for retained products of conception, hysterectomy, and even mortality. When diagnosed in the antepartum or peripartum period, practitioners must take into account minimizing adverse consequences to both the fetus/neonate as well as the mother. Neonatal outcomes vary as widely as the placental pathology outlined in this chapter and depend both on the EGA at diagnosis, severity of the pathology, duration, fetal attributes, as well as peripartum events.

Through the course of this chapter intrinsic and extrinsic placental abnormalities and their clinical correlates have been described. Hopefully, this chapter provided you with an overview of the complex processes of abnormal placentation in relation to real-world outcomes, and will allow you to better understand the following chapters in this book.

Acknowledgements

The author would like to thank the contributions of Rosa Montoya, RN, as well as the indispensable tutelage and mentorship of Martin Gimovsky, MD and Munir Nazir, MD. Writing this book chapter would not have been possible without their prior and continued support, guidance, and love of medicine.

Conflict of interest

The author denies any conflicts of interest associated with this publication.

Future investigation

As medical practitioners, our current prenatal toolkit for treating placental malfunctions is limited, with the main tool being increased fetal surveillance, and when things go awry, the definitive intervention is delivery of the fetus. Until more is known regarding placental pathology and we develop methods for preventing, modifying, treating, or possibly even reversing the pathology, then expedited, and often preterm, delivery with its associated sequellae remains our principal method of therapy. Scientific investigation carries on at a fevered pace, with new findings piecing together the complex biological nature of this fascinating organ. It is this author's hope that during his lifetime, new insights into the placenta on molecular, genetic, physiologic, anatomic, and clinical levels will lead to fetal interventions which thereby decrease the iatrogenic preterm birth rate, and will permit affected pregnancies to progress closer to term in their natural environment.

Appendices and nomenclature

ADAM	amniotic deformity adhesion mutilation sequence
AROM	artificial rupture of membranes
CAM	cellular adhesion molecule
CHTN	chronic hypertension
DIC	disseminated intravascular coagulation
EFW	estimated fetal weight
EGA	estimated gestational age
FFN	fetal fibronectin
HIF	hypoxia inducible factor
IUFD	intrauterine fetal demise
IUGR	intrauterine growth retardation
IVF	in vitro fertilization

MMP	matrix metalloproteinase
MTX	methotrexate
NPV	negative predictive value
NRFHT	non-reassuring fetal heart tracing
PAS	placenta accreta sequence
PlGF	placental growth factor
PPROM	preterm premature rupture of membranes
PPV	positive predictive value
PTL	preterm labor
RCT	randomized controlled trial
sFlt1	soluble FMS-like tyrosine kinase 1
SGA	small for gestational age
SUA	single umbilical artery
iSUA	isolated single uterine artery
SNP	single nucleotide polymorphism
SROM	spontaneous rupture of membranes
TAH	total abdominal hysterectomy
TGF-B1	transforming growth factor-B1
VEGF	vascular endothelial growth factor

Author details

Alexander L. Juusela
Department of Obstetrics and Gynecology, Newark Beth Israel Medical Center, Newark, United States of America

*Address all correspondence to: alex.l.juusela@gmail.com

References

[1] Richardson S, Khandeparker RV, Pellerin P. Amniotic constriction band: A report of two cases with unique clinical presentations. Journal of the Korean Association of Oral and Maxillofacial Surgeons. 2017;**43**:171-177

[2] Madan S, Chaudhuri Z. Amniotic band syndrome: A review of 2 cases. Ophthalmic Plastic & Reconstructive Surgery. Jul/Aug 2018;**34**(4):e110-e113

[3] Martinez-Frias ML. Epidemiological characteristics of amniotic band sequence (ABS) and body wall complex (BWC): Are they two different entities? American Journal of Medical Genetics. 1997;**73**:176-179

[4] Devi PL, Cicy PJ, Thambi R, Poothiode U. Significance of fibrotic bands in utero–amniotic band sequence with limb body wall complex: A rare case of fetal autopsy. Indian Journal of Pathology & Microbiology. 2015;**58**:528-530

[5] Davies BR, Gimenez-Scherer JA. Comparison of the amniotic band disruption complex with acardiac twins does not support its vascular origin. Fetal and Pediatric Pathology. 2007;**26**:87-99

[6] Barzilay E, Harel Y, Haas J, et al. Prenatal diagnosis of amniotic band syndrome—Risk factors and ultrasonic signs. The Journal of Maternal-Fetal & Neonatal Medicine. 2015;**28**:281-283

[7] Becerra-Solano LE, Castaneda-Cisneros G, Corona-Rivera JR, et al. Severe craniofacial involvement due to amniotic band sequence. Fetal and Pediatric Pathology. 2018;**37**:27-37

[8] Belfort MA, Whitehead WE, Ball R, et al. Fetoscopic amniotic band release in a case of Chorioamniotic separation: An innovative new technique. American Journal of Perinatology Reports. 2016;**6**:e222-e225

[9] Chiu DTW, Patel A, Sakamoto S, Chu A. The impact of microsurgery on congenital hand anomalies associated with amniotic band syndrome. Plastic and Reconstructive Surgery—Global Open. 2018;**6**:e1657

[10] Cortez-Ortega C, Garrocho-Rangel JA, Flores-Velazquez J, et al. Management of the amniotic band syndrome with cleft palate: Literature review and report of a case. Case Reports in Dentistry. 2017;**2017**:7620416

[11] Kruszka P, Uwineza A, Mutesa L, et al. Limb body wall complex, amniotic band sequence, or new syndrome caused by mutation in IQ motif containing K (IQCK)? Molecular Genetics & Genomic Medicine. 2015;**3**:424-432

[12] Shah KH, Shah H. A rare combination of amniotic constriction band with osteogenesis imperfecta. BML Case Reports. 11 Nov 2015;**2015**. DOI: 10.1136/bcr-2015-212400

[13] Philipp T, Kalousek DK. Amnion rupture sequence in a first trimester missed abortion. Prenatal Diagnosis. 2001;**21**:835-838

[14] Gajzer DC, Hirzel AC, Saigal G, Rojas CP, Rodriguez MM. Possible genetic origin of limb-body wall complex. Fetal and Pediatric Pathology. 2015;**34**:257-270

[15] Bhat A, Ilyas M, Dev G. Prenatal sonographic diagnosis of limb-body wall complex: Case series of a rare congenital anomaly. Radiology Case Reports. 2016;**11**:116-120

[16] Orioli IM, Ribeiro MG, Castilla EE. Clinical and epidemiological studies

of amniotic deformity, adhesion, and mutilation (ADAM) sequence in a South American (ECLAMC) population. American Journal of Medical Genetics. Part A. 2003;**118A**:135-145

[17] Bijok J, Massalska D, Kucinska-Chahwan A, et al. Complex malformations involving the fetal body wall—Definition and classification issues. Prenatal Diagnosis. 2017;**37**:1033-1039

[18] Mandrekar SR, Amoncar S, Banaulikar S, Sawant V, Pinto RG. Omphalocele, exstrophy of cloaca, imperforate anus and spinal defect (OEIS complex) with overlapping features of body stalk anomaly (limb body wall complex). Indian Journal of Human Genetics. 2014;**20**:195-198

[19] Kim A, Economidis MA, Stohl HE. Placental abruption after amnioreduction for polyhydramnios caused by chorioangioma. BML Case Reports. 5 Mar 2018. DOI: 10.1136/bcr-2017-222399

[20] Voon HY, Amin R, Kok JL, Tan KS. Call for caution: Neonatal portal vein thrombosis following enbucrilate embolization of placental chorioangioma. Fetal Diagnosis and Therapy. 2018;**43**:77-80

[21] Cheng YK, Yu SC, So PL, Leung TY. Ultrasound-guided percutaneous embolisation of placental chorioangioma using cyanoacrylate. Fetal Diagnosis and Therapy. 2017;**41**:76-79

[22] Papaioannou GK, Evangelinakis N, Kourtis P, Konstantinidou A, Papantoniou N. Giant chorioangioma treated with interstitial laser. Ultrasound in Obstetrics & Gynecology. Aug 2018;**52**(2):280-281

[23] Suzuki S. Antenatal screening for circumvallate placenta. Journal of Medical Ultrasonics (2001). 2008;**35**:71-73

[24] Sharma N, Das R, Salam S, Jethani R, Singh AS. Coexistent circumvallate placenta and battledore insertion of umbilical cord resulting in grave obstetric outcome: A case report. Journal of Reproduction & Infertility. 2017;**18**:390-392

[25] Suzuki S. Clinical significance of pregnancies with circumvallate placenta. The Journal of Obstetrics and Gynaecology Research. 2008;**34**:51-54

[26] Taniguchi H, Aoki S, Sakamaki K, et al. Circumvallate placenta: Associated clinical manifestations and complications—A retrospective study. Obstetrics and Gynecology International. 2014;**2014**:986230

[27] Puvabanditsin S, Garrow E, Bhatt M, et al. Four-vessel umbilical cord associated with multiple congenital anomalies: A case report and literature review. Fetal and Pediatric Pathology. 2011;**30**:98-105

[28] Perez-Cosio C, Sheiner E, Abramowicz JS. Four-vessel umbilical cord: Not always a dire prognosis. Journal of Ultrasound in Medicine. 2008;**27**:1389-1391

[29] Schimmel MS, Eidelman AI. Supernumerary umbilical vein resulting in a four-vessel umbilical cord. American Journal of Perinatology. 1998;**15**:299-301

[30] Ebbing C, Kiserud T, Johnsen SL, Albrechtsen S, Rasmussen S. Prevalence, risk factors and outcomes of velamentous and marginal cord insertions: A population-based study of 634,741 pregnancies. PLoS One. 2013;**8**:e70380

[31] Ebbing C, Kiserud T, Johnsen SL, Albrechtsen S, Rasmussen S. Third

stage of labor risks in velamentous and marginal cord insertion: A population-based study. Acta Obstetricia et Gynecologica Scandinavica. 2015;**94**:878-883

[32] Kent EM, Breathnach FM, Gillan JE, et al. Placental cord insertion and birthweight discordance in twin pregnancies: Results of the national prospective ESPRiT study. American Journal of Obstetrics and Gynecology. 2011;**205**:376.e1-376.e7

[33] Pereira N, Yao R, Guilfoil DS, Richard SD, Plante LA. Placenta membranacea with placenta accreta: Radiologic diagnosis and clinical implications. Prenatal Diagnosis. 2013;**33**:1293-1296

[34] Ravangard SF, Henderson K, Fuller K. Placenta membranacea. Archives of Gynecology and Obstetrics. 2013;**288**:709-712

[35] Ekoukou D, Ng Wing Tin L, Nere MB, Bourdet O, Elalaoui Y, Bazin C. Placenta membranacea. Review of the literature, a case report. Journal de Gynécologie Obstétrique et Biologie de la Reproduction (Paris). 1995;**24**:189-193

[36] Prucka S, Clemens M, Craven C, McPherson E. Single umbilical artery: What does it mean for the fetus? A case-control analysis of pathologically ascertained cases. Genetics in Medicine. 2004;**6**:54-57

[37] Friebe-Hoffmann U, Hiltmann A, Friedl TWP, et al. Prenatally diagnosed single umbilical artery (SUA)—Retrospective analysis of 1169 fetuses. Ultraschall in der Medizin. 28 Mar 2018. DOI: 10.1055/s-0043-123463 [Epub ahead of print]

[38] Gurram P, Figueroa R, Sipusic E, Kuhnly N, Clark S, Janicki MB. Isolated single umbilical artery and fetal echocardiography: A 25-year experience at a tertiary Care City hospital. Journal of Ultrasound in Medicine. 2018;**37**:463-468

[39] Battarbee AN, Palatnik A, Ernst LM, Grobman WA. Placental abnormalities associated with isolated single umbilical artery in small-for-gestational-age births. Placenta. 2017;**59**:9-12

[40] Kim HJ, Kim JH, Chay DB, Park JH, Kim MA. Association of isolated single umbilical artery with perinatal outcomes: Systemic review and meta-analysis. Obstetrics & Gynecology Science. 2017;**60**:266-273

[41] Araujo Junior E, Palma-Dias R, Martins WP, Reidy K, da Silva Costa F. Congenital heart disease and adverse perinatal outcome in fetuses with confirmed isolated single functioning umbilical artery. Journal of Obstetrics and Gynaecology. 2015;**35**:85-87

[42] Iqbal S, Raiz I. Isolated single umbilical artery in twin pregnancies and its adverse pregnancy outcomes—A case report and review of literature. Journal of Clinical and Diagnostic Research. 2015;**9**:AD01-AD04

[43] Arcos-Machancoses JV, Marin-Reina P, Romaguera-Salort E, Garcia-Camunas Y, Perez-Aytes A, Vento M. Postnatal development of fetuses with a single umbilical artery: Differences between malformed and non-malformed infants. World Journal of Pediatrics. 2015;**11**:61-66

[44] Ruiter L, Ravelli AC, De Graaf IM, Mol BW, Pajkrt E. Incidence and recurrence rate of placental abruption: A longitudinal linked national cohort study in the Netherlands. American Journal of Obstetrics and Gynecology. 2015;**213**:573.e1-573.e8

[45] Bronsteen R, Whitten A, Balasubramanian M, et al. Vasa previa: Clinical presentations, outcomes, and implications for management.

Obstetrics and Gynecology. 2013;**122**:352-357

[46] Sinkin JA, Craig WY, Jones M, Pinette MG, Wax JR. Perinatal outcomes associated with isolated velamentous cord insertion in singleton and twin pregnancies. Journal of Ultrasound in Medicine. 2018;**37**:471-478

[47] Maymon R, Melcer Y, Tovbin J, Pekar-Zlotin M, Smorgick N, Jauniaux E. The rate of cervical length shortening in the management of vasa previa. Journal of Ultrasound in Medicine. 2018;**37**:717-723

[48] Smorgick N, Tovbin Y, Ushakov F, et al. Is neonatal risk from vasa previa preventable? The 20-year experience from a single medical center. Journal of Clinical Ultrasound. 2010;**38**:118-122

[49] Ebbing C, Johnsen SL, Albrechtsen S, Sunde ID, Vekseth C, Rasmussen S. Velamentous or marginal cord insertion and the risk of spontaneous preterm birth, prelabor rupture of the membranes, and anomalous cord length, a population-based study. Acta Obstetricia et Gynecologica Scandinavica. 2017;**96**:78-85

[50] de Los Reyes S, Henderson J, Eke AC. A systematic review and meta-analysis of velamentous cord insertion among singleton pregnancies and the risk of preterm delivery. International Journal of Gynaecology and Obstetrics. 2018;**142**:9-14

[51] Stulberg DB, Cain LR, Dahlquist I, Lauderdale DS. Ectopic pregnancy rates and racial disparities in the Medicaid population, 2004-2008. Fertility and Sterility. 2014;**102**:1671-1676

[52] Hoover RN, Hyer M, Pfeiffer RM, et al. Adverse health outcomes in women exposed in utero to diethylstilbestrol. The New England Journal of Medicine. 2011;**365**:1304-1314

[53] Bouyer J, Coste J, Fernandez H, Pouly JL, Job-Spira N. Sites of ectopic pregnancy: A 10 year population-based study of 1800 cases. Human Reproduction. 2002;**17**:3224-3230

[54] Cho YK, Henning S, Harkins G. Broad ligament ectopic pregnancy after bilateral tubal ligation. Journal of Minimally Invasive Gynecology. 2018;**25**:314-315

[55] Committee on Practice B-G. ACOG practice bulletin No. 191: Tubal ectopic pregnancy. Obstetrics and Gynecology. 2018;**131**:e65-e77

[56] Huang YT, Liang IT, Wang CJ. Tubo-omental ectopic pregnancy. Journal of Minimally Invasive Gynecology. 2018;**25**: 569-570

[57] Frates MC, Benson CB, Doubilet PM, et al. Cervical ectopic pregnancy: Results of conservative treatment. Radiology. 1994;**191**:773-775

[58] Mahgoub S, Gabriele V, Faller E, et al. Cesarean scar ectopic pregnancy: Laparoscopic resection and Total scar dehiscence repair. Journal of Minimally Invasive Gynecology. 2018;**25**:297-298

[59] Creanga AA, Shapiro-Mendoza CK, Bish CL, Zane S, Berg CJ, Callaghan WM. Trends in ectopic pregnancy mortality in the United States: 1980-2007. Obstetrics and Gynecology. 2011;**117**:837-843

[60] Creanga AA, Syverson C, Seed K, Callaghan WM. Pregnancy-related mortality in the United States, 2011-2013. Obstetrics and Gynecology. 2017;**130**:366-373

[61] Lin S, Yang R, Chi H, et al. Increased incidence of ectopic pregnancy after in vitro fertilization in women with decreased ovarian reserve. Oncotarget. 2017;**8**:14570-14575

[62] Marion LL, Meeks GR. Ectopic pregnancy: History, incidence, epidemiology, and risk factors. Clinical Obstetrics and Gynecology. 2012;**55**:376-386

[63] Coste J, Bouyer J, Ughetto S, et al. Ectopic pregnancy is again on the increase. Recent trends in the incidence of ectopic pregnancies in France (1992-2002). Human Reproduction. 2004;**19**:2014-2018

[64] Faiz AS, Ananth CV. Etiology and risk factors for placenta previa: An overview and meta-analysis of observational studies. The Journal of Maternal-Fetal & Neonatal Medicine. 2003;**13**:175-190

[65] Cresswell JA, Ronsmans C, Calvert C, Filippi V. Prevalence of placenta praevia by world region: A systematic review and meta-analysis. Tropical Medicine & International Health. 2013;**18**:712-724

[66] Usta IM, Hobeika EM, Musa AA, Gabriel GE, Nassar AH. Placenta previa-accreta: Risk factors and complications. American Journal of Obstetrics and Gynecology. 2005;**193**:1045-1049

[67] Ananth CV, Smulian JC, Vintzileos AM. The association of placenta previa with history of cesarean delivery and abortion: A metaanalysis. American Journal of Obstetrics and Gynecology. 1997;**177**:1071-1078

[68] Getahun D, Oyelese Y, Salihu HM, Ananth CV. Previous cesarean delivery and risks of placenta previa and placental abruption. Obstetrics and Gynecology. 2006;**107**:771-778

[69] Gilliam M, Rosenberg D, Davis F. The likelihood of placenta previa with greater number of cesarean deliveries and higher parity. Obstetrics and Gynecology. 2002;**99**:976-980

[70] Weis MA, Harper LM, Roehl KA, Odibo AO, Cahill AG. Natural history of placenta previa in twins. Obstetrics and Gynecology. 2012;**120**:753-758

[71] Chantraine F, Blacher S, Berndt S, et al. Abnormal vascular architecture at the placental-maternal interface in placenta increta. American Journal of Obstetrics and Gynecology. 2012;**207**:188.e1-188.e9

[72] Chantraine F, Braun T, Gonser M, Henrich W, Tutschek B. Prenatal diagnosis of abnormally invasive placenta reduces maternal peripartum hemorrhage and morbidity. Acta Obstetricia et Gynecologica Scandinavica. 2013;**92**:439-444

[73] Cohen M, Wuillemin C, Irion O, Bischof P. Role of decidua in trophoblastic invasion. Neuro Endocrinology Letters. 2010;**31**:193-197

[74] Jauniaux E, Collins S, Burton GJ. Placenta accreta spectrum: Pathophysiology and evidence-based anatomy for prenatal ultrasound imaging. American Journal of Obstetrics and Gynecology. 2018;**218**:75-87

[75] Cho FN, Liu CB, Li JY, Yu KJ, Chen SN. Prominent decidual vasculature overlying the internal cervical os: An entity potentially leading to acute life-threatening antepartum hemorrhage. Journal of the Chinese Medical Association. 2010;**73**:216-218

[76] Wehrum MJ, Buhimschi IA, Salafia C, et al. Accreta complicating complete placenta previa is characterized by reduced systemic levels of vascular endothelial growth factor and by epithelial-to-mesenchymal transition of the invasive trophoblast. American Journal of Obstetrics and Gynecology. 2011;**204**:411.e1-411.e11

[77] Rosen T. Placenta accreta and cesarean scar pregnancy: Overlooked

costs of the rising cesarean section rate. Clinics in Perinatology. 2008;**35**: 519-529 x

[78] Wu S, Kocherginsky M, Hibbard JU. Abnormal placentation: Twenty-year analysis. American Journal of Obstetrics and Gynecology. 2005;**192**:1458-1461

[79] Glaze S, Ekwalanga P, Roberts G, et al. Peripartum hysterectomy: 1999 to 2006. Obstetrics and Gynecology. 2008;**111**:732-738

[80] Duzyj CM, Buhimschi IA, Laky CA, et al. Extravillous trophoblast invasion in placenta accreta is associated with differential local expression of angiogenic and growth factors: A cross-sectional study. British Journal of Obstetrics and Gynaecology. Oct 2018;**125**(11):1441-1448

[81] Panigrahi AK, Yeaton-Massey A, Bakhtary S, et al. A standardized approach for transfusion medicine support in patients with morbidly adherent placenta. Anesthesia and Analgesia. 2017;**125**:603-608

[82] Flood KM, Said S, Geary M, Robson M, Fitzpatrick C, Malone FD. Changing trends in peripartum hysterectomy over the last 4 decades. American Journal of Obstetrics and Gynecology. 2009;**200**:632.e1-632.e6

[83] Imudia AN, Awonuga AO, Dbouk T, et al. Incidence, trends, risk factors, indications for, and complications associated with cesarean hysterectomy: A 17-year experience from a single institution. Archives of Gynecology and Obstetrics. 2009;**280**:619-623

[84] Clark SL, Koonings PP, Phelan JP. Placenta previa/accreta and prior cesarean section. Obstetrics and Gynecology. 1985;**66**:89-92

[85] Read JA, Cotton DB, Miller FC. Placenta accreta: Changing clinical aspects and outcome. Obstetrics and Gynecology. 1980;**56**:31-34

[86] Silver RM, Landon MB, Rouse DJ, et al. Maternal morbidity associated with multiple repeat cesarean deliveries. Obstetrics and Gynecology. 2006;**107**(6):1226-1232

[87] Mehrabadi A, Hutcheon JA, Liu S, et al. Contribution of placenta accreta to the incidence of postpartum hemorrhage and severe postpartum hemorrhage. Obstetrics and Gynecology. 2015;**125**:814-821

[88] Matsubara S, Kuwata T, Usui R, et al. Important surgical measures and techniques at cesarean hysterectomy for placenta previa accreta. Acta Obstetricia et Gynecologica Scandinavica. 2013;**92**:372-377

[89] Timor-Tritsch IE, Monteagudo A. Unforeseen consequences of the increasing rate of cesarean deliveries: Early placenta accreta and cesarean scar pregnancy. A review. American Journal of Obstetrics and Gynecology. 2012;**207**:14-29

[90] Esakoff TF, Sparks TN, Kaimal AJ, et al. Diagnosis and morbidity of placenta accreta. Ultrasound in Obstetrics & Gynecology. 2011;**37**:324-327

[91] Warshak CR, Eskander R, Hull AD, et al. Accuracy of ultrasonography and magnetic resonance imaging in the diagnosis of placenta accreta. Obstetrics and Gynecology. 2006;**108**:573-581

[92] Rac MW, Dashe JS, Wells CE, Moschos E, McIntire DD, Twickler DM. Ultrasound predictors of placental invasion: The placenta Accreta index. American Journal of Obstetrics and Gynecology. 2015;**212**:343.e1-343.e7

[93] Elhawary TM, Dabees NL, Youssef MA. Diagnostic value of ultrasonography and magnetic resonance imaging in pregnant women at risk for placenta accreta. The Journal of Maternal-Fetal & Neonatal Medicine. 2013;**26**:1443-1449

[94] Sentilhes L, Ambroselli C, Kayem G, et al. Maternal outcome after conservative treatment of placenta accreta. Obstetrics and Gynecology. 2010;**115**:526-534

[95] Committee on Obstetric P. Committee opinion no. 529: placenta accreta. Obstetrics and Gynecology. 2012;**120**:207-211

[96] English D, Verma U, Yasin S. Conservative management of a 20-week cervical ectopic pregnancy with placenta percreta. Archives of Gynecology and Obstetrics. 2013;**288**:225-228

[97] Verma U, Maggiorotto F. Conservative management of second-trimester cervical ectopic pregnancy with placenta percreta. Fertility and Sterility. 2007;**87**:697.e13-697.e16

[98] Tariq A, O'Rourke M, Carstens SJ, Totten VY. Intra-abdominal rupture of a live cervical pregnancy with placenta Accreta but without vaginal bleeding. Clinical Practice and Cases in Emergency Medicine. 2018;**2**:116-120

[99] Large MJ, Wetendorf M, Lanz RB, et al. The epidermal growth factor receptor critically regulates endometrial function during early pregnancy. PLoS Genetics. 2014;**10**:e1004451

[100] Lee JH, Kim TH, Oh SJ, et al. Signal transducer and activator of transcription-3 (Stat3) plays a critical role in implantation via progesterone receptor in uterus. The FASEB Journal. 2013;**27**:2553-2563

[101] Lessey BA, Albelda S, Buck CA, et al. Distribution of integrin cell adhesion molecules in endometrial cancer. The American Journal of Pathology. 1995;**146**:717-726

[102] Jia Y, Li T, Huang X, et al. Dysregulated DNA methyltransferase 3A upregulates IGFBP5 to suppress trophoblast cell migration and invasion in preeclampsia. Hypertension. 2017;**69**:356-366

[103] Zhu Y, Lu H, Huo Z, et al. MicroRNA-16 inhibits feto-maternal angiogenesis and causes recurrent spontaneous abortion by targeting vascular endothelial growth factor. Scientific Reports. 2016;**6**:35536

[104] Soygur B, Moore H. Expression of Syncytin 1 (HERV-W), in the preimplantation human blastocyst, embryonic stem cells and trophoblast cells derived in vitro. Human Reproduction. 2016;**31**:1455-1461

[105] Chen J, Khalil RA. Matrix metalloproteinases in normal pregnancy and preeclampsia. Progress in Molecular Biology and Translational Science. 2017;**148**:87-165

[106] Lessey BA, Castelbaum AJ, Sawin SW, Sun J. Integrins as markers of uterine receptivity in women with primary unexplained infertility. Fertility and Sterility. 1995;**63**:535-542

[107] Lessey BA. Adhesion molecules and implantation. Journal of Reproductive Immunology. 2002;**55**:101-112

[108] Lessey BA, Gui Y, Apparao KB, Young SL, Mulholland J. Regulated expression of heparin-binding EGF-like growth factor (HB-EGF) in the human endometrium: A potential paracrine role during implantation. Molecular Reproduction and Development. 2002;**62**:446-455

[109] Wikstrom AK, Larsson A, Eriksson UJ, Nash P, Norden-Lindeberg S, Olovsson M. Placental growth

factor and soluble FMS-like tyrosine kinase-1 in early-onset and late-onset preeclampsia. Obstetrics and Gynecology. 2007;**109**:1368-1374

[110] March MI, Geahchan C, Wenger J, et al. Circulating Angiogenic factors and the risk of adverse outcomes among Haitian women with preeclampsia. PLoS One. 2015;**10**:e0126815

[111] Kenchegowda D, Natale B, Lemus MA, Natale DR, Fisher SA. Inactivation of maternal Hif-1alpha at mid-pregnancy causes placental defects and deficits in oxygen delivery to the fetal organs under hypoxic stress. Developmental Biology. 2017;**422**:171-185

[112] Norwitz ER. Defective implantation and placentation: Laying the blueprint for pregnancy complications. Reproductive Biomedicine Online. 2006;**13**:591-599

[113] Lim KH, Zhou Y, Janatpour M, et al. Human cytotrophoblast differentiation/invasion is abnormal in pre-eclampsia. The American Journal of Pathology. 1997;**151**:1809-1818

[114] Chigusa Y, Kishore AH, Mogami H, Word RA. Nrf2 activation inhibits effects of thrombin in human amnion cells and thrombin-induced preterm birth in mice. The Journal of Clinical Endocrinology and Metabolism. 2016;**101**:2612-2621

[115] Mogami H, Kishore AH, Shi H, Keller PW, Akgul Y, Word RA. Fetal fibronectin signaling induces matrix metalloproteases and cyclooxygenase-2 (COX-2) in amnion cells and preterm birth in mice. The Journal of Biological Chemistry. 2013;**288**:1953-1966

[116] Rowe TF, King LA, MacDonald PC, Casey ML. Tissue inhibitor of metalloproteinase-1 and tissue inhibitor of metalloproteinase-2 expression in human amnion mesenchymal and epithelial cells. American Journal of Obstetrics and Gynecology. 1997;**176**:915-921

[117] Nagy S, Bush M, Stone J, Lapinski RH, Gardo S. Clinical significance of subchorionic and retroplacental hematomas detected in the first trimester of pregnancy. Obstetrics and Gynecology. 2003;**102**:94-100

[118] Zhou J, Wu M, Wang B, et al. The effect of first trimester subchorionic hematoma on pregnancy outcomes in patients underwent IVF/ICSI treatment. The Journal of Maternal-Fetal & Neonatal Medicine. 2017;**30**:406-410

[119] Ananth CV, Keyes KM, Hamilton A, et al. An international contrast of rates of placental abruption: An age-period-cohort analysis. PLoS One. 2015;**10**:e0125246

[120] Tikkanen M. Placental abruption: Epidemiology, risk factors and consequences. Acta Obstetricia et Gynecologica Scandinavica. 2011;**90**:140-149

[121] Ananth CV, Getahun D, Peltier MR, Smulian JC. Placental abruption in term and preterm gestations: Evidence for heterogeneity in clinical pathways. Obstetrics and Gynecology. 2006;**107**:785-792

[122] Elsasser DA, Ananth CV, Prasad V, Vintzileos AM. New Jersey—Placental abruption study I. Diagnosis of placental abruption: Relationship between clinical and histopathological findings. European Journal of Obstetrics, Gynecology, and Reproductive Biology. 2010;**148**: 125-130

[123] Tuuli MG, Norman SM, Odibo AO, Macones GA, Cahill AG. Perinatal outcomes in women with subchorionic hematoma: A systematic review and meta-analysis. Obstetrics and Gynecology. 2011;**117**:1205-1212

[124] Seki H, Kuromaki K, Takeda S, Kinoshita K. Persistent subchorionic hematoma with clinical symptoms until delivery. International Journal of Gynaecology and Obstetrics. 1998;**63**:123-128

[125] Ananth CV, Savitz DA, Williams MA. Placental abruption and its association with hypertension and prolonged rupture of membranes: A methodologic review and meta-analysis. Obstetrics and Gynecology. 1996;**88**:309-318

[126] Pariente G, Wiznitzer A, Sergienko R, Mazor M, Holcberg G, Sheiner E. Placental abruption: Critical analysis of risk factors and perinatal outcomes. The Journal of Maternal-Fetal & Neonatal Medicine. 2011;**24**:698-702

[127] Rasmussen S, Irgens LM, Dalaker K. A history of placental dysfunction and risk of placental abruption. Paediatric and Perinatal Epidemiology. 1999;**13**:9-21

[128] Kobayashi A, Minami S, Tanizaki Y, et al. Adverse perinatal and neonatal outcomes in patients with chronic abruption-oligohydramnios sequence. The Journal of Obstetrics and Gynaecology Research. 2014;**40**:1618-1624

[129] Kurata Y, Kido A, Minamiguchi S, Kondoh E, Togashi K. MRI findings of chronic abruption-oligohydramnios sequence (CAOS): Report of three cases. Abdominal Radiology (NY). 2017;**42**:1839-1844

[130] Rasmussen S, Irgens LM, Dalaker K. Outcome of pregnancies subsequent to placental abruption: A risk assessment. Acta Obstetricia et Gynecologica Scandinavica. 2000;**79**:496-501

[131] Rasmussen S, Irgens LM. Occurrence of placental abruption in relatives. British Journal of Obstetrics and Gynaecology. 2009;**116**:693-699

[132] Toivonen S, Heinonen S, Anttila M, Kosma VM, Saarikoski S. Obstetric prognosis after placental abruption. Fetal Diagnosis and Therapy. 2004;**19**:336-341

[133] Tikkanen M, Nuutila M, Hiilesmaa V, Paavonen J, Ylikorkala O. Prepregnancy risk factors for placental abruption. Acta Obstetricia et Gynecologica Scandinavica. 2006;**85**:40-44

[134] Gris JC, Chauleur C, Faillie JL, et al. Enoxaparin for the secondary prevention of placental vascular complications in women with abruptio placentae. The pilot randomised controlled NOH-AP trial. Thrombosis and Haemostasis. 2010;**104**:771-779

Section 2

Clinical Application

Chapter 2

Miscarriage and Maternal Health

John D. Ojule and Rosemary N. Ogu

Abstract

Miscarriage also known as spontaneous abortion is the termination of pregnancy before the age of fetal viability or expulsion of fetus or embryo weighing less than 500g. It occurs naturally without any human intervention and complicates about 15–20% pregnancies globally. The age of fetal viability varies from country to country depending on the level of technological development and fetal salvage rate. The age of fetal viability in Norway is 16 weeks, in Australia its 20 weeks, 24 weeks in the UK, 26 weeks in Spain and Italy while in Nigeria the age of fetal viability is 28 weeks of gestation. Causes of miscarriage include morphologic/genetic/chromosomal abnormalities, immunological and endocrine factors, structural uterine anomalies, cervical incompetence, maternal infections and toxins. It is classified into threatened miscarriage, inevitable miscarriage, incomplete miscarriage, septic miscarriage, missed miscarriage and complete miscarriage. Miscarriage has profound and tremendous psychologic and emotional effects on mothers before or during subsequent gestations. Every effort must be made to show understanding and empathy.

Keywords: pregnancy loss, maternal health, miscarriage, women's health, introduction

1. Introduction

Miscarriage also known as spontaneous abortion is the termination of pregnancy before the age of fetal viability or expulsion of fetus or embryo weighing less than 500g. It occurs naturally without any human intervention and complicates about 15–20% pregnancies globally. The age of fetal viability varies from country to country depending on the level of technological development and fetal salvage rate. The age of fetal viability in Norway is 16 weeks, in Australia its 20 weeks, 24 weeks in the UK, 26 weeks in Spain and Italy while in Nigeria the age of fetal viability is 28 weeks of gestation. Causes of miscarriage include morphologic/genetic/chromosomal abnormalities, immunological and endocrine factors, structural uterine anomalies, cervical incompetence, maternal infections and toxins. Miscarriage can be classified into threatened miscarriage, inevitable miscarriage, incomplete miscarriage, septic miscarriage, missed miscarriage, complete miscarriage and recurrent miscarriage. It profoundly affects the women. This chapter methodology derives from a synthesis of the available literature under the MESH search term miscarriage and focus group discussion of women attending a tertiary health facility in Southern Nigeria.

2. Miscarriage and maternal morbidity

Miscarriage can profoundly affect the health and wellbeing of the mother, either from the complications of the process itself or from the complications arising from the treatment and management of the condition or both depending on the stage of the pregnancy, the abortion type, the management instituted, the facility, the skill/expertise and quality of the care giver and the mother's pre-pregnancy/pre-miscarriage health condition.

The complications can arise early, during or just after the process or manifest much later following the abortion process, also depending on several factors.

2.1 Early morbidities

2.1.1 Hemorrhage

Genital bleeding during or following miscarriage may be slight especially in early 1st trimester, but can also be severe and torrential with disastrous consequences in the second trimester when there is increased risk of placenta retention. This may occur more commonly in the developing countries like Nigeria where mothers may not present to health facilities for optimal management due to ignorance, illiteracy, poverty, non-availability or poor accessibility to health care facilities especially women in remote areas. Even when they do, they may present late to the health facility, at that further complications including severe anemia, sepsis, shock etc. may have set in, worsening maternal health and making management difficult in resource poor setting.

Management entails controlling the bleeding with use of oxytocics and delivery of the placenta by skilled and experienced care provider either by careful controlled cord traction or piece meal removal with sponge holding forceps and antibiotic therapy.

2.1.2 Anemia

Anemia may occur more commonly from hemorrhage or occasionally from sepsis due to hemolysis or both. Management of anemia in developing countries, especially when severe, may be particularly difficult because of the problems enumerated earlier. Even when mothers access health facility, there may not be blood banking services or when available may not be functioning optimally because of endemic problems of electricity and corruption with its negative multiplier effects in sub-Saharan Africa.

2.1.3 Septic incomplete abortion

Incomplete miscarriage occurs when some of the products of conception have been expelled while some are still retained in the uterus. This may cause bleeding which may range from mild to severe, causing blood loss anemia that may require blood transfusion. When bleeding is severe and not properly managed in time, post abortal pituitary necrosis resulting in Sheehan's syndrome may occur, which later causes infertility which causes infertility later.

When some of the products of conception have been expelled and some retained, as may happen at gestational age 10 and above, this becomes substrate for microbial colonization and eventual infection. This infection may become severe causing systemic effects like fever, vomiting and prostration. Long term complications will include Asherman's syndrome, chronic pelvic inflammatory disease, frozen pelvis and infertility as discussed in late maternal morbidities. Septicemia may occur and if not properly managed may result in multiple organ injury with sequelae.

2.1.4 Post-abortal sepsis

Post abortal sepsis usually results from complete miscarriage managed with inadequate or without prophylactic antibiotics. It may also occur if incomplete miscarriage is evacuated in an unhygienic environment or by unskilled care provider.

Mothers may present days, weeks or even months following miscarriage with varying degrees of abdominal pain, vaginal discharge or subfertility. These can be distressing and negatively affected maternal health. This can lead to loss of man hours in work place, school resulting in economic loss. Marital disharmony may also arise from infertility especially in sub-Saharan Africa where high premium is placed on child bearing. There is also a huge burden on health care delivery occasioned by these health challenges.

2.1.5 Shock

Shock could be hypovolemic or cardiogenic from massive hemorrhage or even septic from Gram negative sepsis with its very high mortality rate.

2.1.6 Organ injury

Though more common with induced abortion, uterine perforation can also occur following curettage or manual vacuum aspiration in the management of incomplete miscarriage. In acute state this can cause acute abdomen and may require hospitalization and even laparotomy. This affects maternal health in the short run and even in the long run depending on the nature and severity of the injury.

Bladder and injury to the intestinal injuries have also been reported. A couple times in the Accident and Emergency department of the University of Port Harcourt Teaching Hospital, Port Harcourt, Nigeria, patients have presented with large intestine protruding from the introitus through the uterus following manual vacuum aspiration for incomplete miscarriage done by unskilled health care provider.

More often, these will require laparotomy, repair of uterine perforation, bowel resection and anastomosis.

Bladder injury may even be more devastating when genito-urinary fistula manifest with continuous leakage of urine, with its accompanying morbidities- vulva excoriations/ itching, disgusting and nauseating offensive ammoniacal smell, social stigma, subfertility and sometimes marital disharmony and divorce. The emotional and psychological trauma is unparalleled.

2.2 Late morbidities

Some morbidities may not manifest immediately or early but become apparent months or even years following miscarriage or treatment of miscarriage.

2.2.1 PID/frozen pelvis

Pelvic inflammatory disease may complicate poorly treated incomplete miscarriage. This may subsequently lead to chronic PID especially in resource poor settings where people resort to self-management of the condition using sometimes unorthodox methods. They may present with chronic pelvic pain, dysmenorrhea or even amenorrhea depending on the severity, dyspareunia, chronic vaginal discharge and or low back pain. In some instances they may develop tubo-ovarian mass or abscess resulting in frozen pelvis. All these no doubt will negatively impact maternal health.

2.2.2 Asherman's syndrome/infertility

Oligomenorrhea, amenorrhea and subfertility constitute Asherman's syndrome. This results from scarring occasioned by healing from endometritis or healing from overzealous curettage in management of incomplete miscarriage.

2.3 Psychological/emotional morbidities

Prior miscarriage or even just perception of miscarriage can have profound and tremendous psychologic and emotional effects on mothers before or during subsequent gestations.

Studies have shown that compared to women without prior miscarriage, women with previous history of miscarriage had greater state anxiety in the second and third trimesters. Having a living child did not buffer state anxiety in women with a prior miscarriage. Attention to patterns of distress can contribute to delivery of appropriate support resources to women experiencing pregnancy after miscarriage and may help reduce risk for stress-related outcomes.

Just like other stressful experiences, the effects of miscarriage vary considerably across individuals [1], but for many women, miscarriage can be a tragic, and life-altering experience [2] and results in significant suffering [3, 4]. In the last 20 years, research on the emotional and psychological impact of miscarriage has grown, including studies of women who have experienced miscarriage exclusively and mixed-sample studies of various types of perinatal loss including miscarriage, stillbirth, and neonatal death, establishing an empirical foundation for understanding the livid experiences of miscarriage. Women who experience miscarriage worry about future pregnancies [4] and may perceive a subsequent pregnancy as especially precious and very desirable [5]. Pregnancy after miscarriage can be experienced as emotionally and psychologically distressing [4, 6]. According to descriptive studies of pregnancy following miscarriage, for some women the subsequent pregnancy is perceived as threatening [7] and involves tremendous vulnerability and anxiety related to uncertainty about its outcome [8].

Researchers who included comparison groups of mothers without a prior history of miscarriage have found that women with a history of miscarriage, experience significantly higher state anxiety, pregnancy-specific anxiety, worry, depression, and less attachment to the subsequent pregnancy than women without prior miscarriage [9, 10].

The most prevalent finding is that pregnancy-specific anxiety is higher in those with prior loss [10, 11], but more generalized distress does not differ significantly between the groups [10, 12] of perinatal loss. It has been demonstrated that pregnancy anxiety decreased significantly over the course of pregnancy [7]. focus group discussion with parturients attending antenatal care in Port Harcourt, Nigeria, revealed similar findings. The psychosomatic stress experienced by women who have had a prior miscarriage is better imagined then experienced. The feeling of being responsible for the loss coupled with the premium placed on childbirth leads to profound anxiety, sadness and depression. Understanding and empathy from healthcare providers and family members aided the recovery process.

3. Conclusion

Miscarriage or even just perception of miscarriage can have profound and tremendous psychologic and emotional effects on mothers before or during subsequent gestations. The associated early and long term complications are devastating for women. Every effort must be made to show understanding and empathy.

Author details

John D. Ojule and Rosemary N. Ogu*
Department of Obstetrics and Gynaecology University of Port Harcourt,
Port Harcourt, Nigeria

*Address all correspondence to: rosemary.ogu@uniport.edu.ng

References

[1] Huffman CS, Schwartz TA, Swanson KM. Couples and miscarriage: The influence of gender and reproductive factors on the impact of miscarriage. Women's Health Issues. 2015;**25**(5):570-578

[2] Radford EJ, Hughes M. Women's experiences of early miscarriage: Implications for nursing care. Journal of Clinical Nursing. 2015;**24**(11-12):1457-1465

[3] San Lazaro Campillo I, Meaney S, McNamara K, O'Donoghue K. Psychological and support interventions to reduce levels of stress, anxiety or depression on women's subsequent pregnancy with a history of miscarriage: An empty systematic review. BMJ Open. 2017;**7**(9):e017802

[4] Geller PA, Kerns D, Klier CM. Anxiety following miscarriage and the subsequent pregnancy. A review of literature and future directions. Journal of Psychosomatic Research. 2004;**56**:35-45

[5] Cannella BL, Yarcheski A, Mahon NE. Meta-analyses of predictors of health practices in pregnant women. Western Journal of Nursing Research;**40**(3):425-446

[6] Bhat A, Infertility BN. Perinatal loss: When the bough breaks. Current Psychiatry Reports. 2016;**18**(3):31

[7] Cote-Arsenault D. Threat appraisal, coping, and emotions across pregnancy subsequent to perinatal loss. Nursing Research. 2007;**56**:108-116

[8] Côté-Arsenault D, Schwartz K, Krowchuk H, McCoy TP. Evidence-based intervention with women pregnant after perinatal loss. MCN: The American Journal of Maternal/Child Nursing. 2014;**39**(3):177

[9] Moore T, Parrish H, Black BP. Interconception care for couples after perinatal loss: A comprehensive review of the literature. The Journal of Perinatal & Neonatal Nursing. 2011;**25**(1):44-51

[10] Cote-Arsenault D. The influence of perinatal loss on anxiety in multigravidas. Journal of Obstetrics, Gynaecologic and Neonatal Nursing. 2003;**32**:623-629

[11] Armstrong D, Hutti M. Pregnancy after perinatal loss: The relationship between anxiety and prenatal attachment. Journal of Obstetrics, Gynecologic and Neonatal Nursing. 1998;**27**:183-189

[12] Franche RI, Mikail SF. The impact of perinatal loss on adjustment to subsequent pregnancy. Social Science and Medicine. 1999;**48**:1613-1623

Chapter 3

Assessment of Fetal Gestational Age in the First Trimester in Normal and Abnormal Pregnancies: Which Sonographic Parameter to Use?

Hong Soo Wong

Abstract

To compare the correlation of various fetal ultrasound parameters to foot length, crown-rump length, and gestational age by date to determine the best estimate at 10–14 completed weeks' gestation and to provide ratios of fetal parameters for assessment of fetal abnormalities in the first trimester. 35 routine obstetric scans were performed at 10–14 completed weeks' gestation for fetal parameters and ratios. The fetal crown-rump length (CRL), biparietal diameter (BPD), head circumference (HC), abdominal circumference (AC), and femur length (FL) showed a linear correlation with the estimated gestational age by date (GA), crown-rump length (CRL), and foot length (FT) ($p < 0.001$), with the least correlation observed with GA and highest with FT. A combination of BPD, HC, AC, and FL correlated best with FT and then CRL and GA ($R^2 = 0.881$, 0.795, and 0.685, respectively, $p < 0.001$). With the addition of CRL, R^2 was 0.859. The ratio of FL/AC and FL/FT to FT, CRL, GA, BPD, and HC increases in an inverse relationship at 10–14 completed weeks' gestation. The combination of BPD, HC, AC, and FL provides a better estimation of gestational age than (and hence may replace) CRL or GA at 10–14 weeks' gestation.

Keywords: ultrasonography, fetus, pregnancy, first trimester, prenatal diagnosis

1. Introduction

The fetal foot is one of the first structures identifiable early in the human embryos. At the end of the fourth week of embryonic development, the limb buds appear as outpouchings from the ventrolateral body wall. At 6 weeks, the terminal portion of the limb buds flattens to form the hand- and footplates and becomes separated from the proximal segment by a circular constriction. It is known that the development of the lower limbs is similar to the upper limbs and lags by only 1–2 days. By 8 weeks (or 56 days), the digital separation is already complete. The fingers and the toes are distinct and separated in the hands and feet [1, 2]. In another word, the fetal hands and feet would be recognizable as distinct formed structures by 8 weeks of embryological development or 10 weeks by the last menstrual period (LMP) according to a 28 day cycle.

About a century ago, Streeter reported a linear correlation between gestational age and foot length in 704 human fetal specimens from around 50 days post-conception until birth [3]. This linear correlation has been confirmed by studies on live fetuses in utero on transabdominal [4–6] or transvaginal scans [7] or on dead fetuses at abortion [8–10] or stillbirth [11, 12], and nomograms have been developed for assessment of fetal gestational age with foot length (FT) from the first trimester to later gestation. Hence, fetal foot length could by itself stand as a proxy for gestational age even in early pregnancy.

Conventionally, crown-rump length (CRL) is used as the reference parameter for assessment of fetal gestational age in the first trimester ultrasound scan [13, 14]. It has been suggested that the ultrasound measurement of the crown-rump length in the embryo or fetus is the most accurate method to establish or confirm gestational age in the first trimester up to 13 + 6 weeks [14]. The use of routine first trimester ultrasound scan has been shown to be associated with a reduction in induction of labor for post-term pregnancy [15]. However, there is little information on the comparison of other fetal parameters including biparietal diameter (BPD), head circumference (HC), abdominal circumference (AC), femur length (FL), and foot length to CRL in the assessment of gestational age in early gestation [16]. This information may be important for the assessment of fetal gestational age in the first trimester and subsequent management of pregnancy.

In order to ascertain the performance of various parameters in assessment of gestational age in the first trimester, in this chapter, the correlation between FT, CRL, and gestational age assessed by date (GA) will be compared from 10 to 14 weeks gestation. The correlation of the other fetal parameters (BPD, HC, AC, and FL) will also be compared to GA, CRL, and FT. Moreover, the ratio of some of these parameters will also be calculated and presented, as the availability of such ratios may be helpful when fetal abnormality is suspected on ultrasound examination in early pregnancy [17–19].

2. Method and material

Transabdominal ultrasound examination was performed as a part of routine antenatal assessment for women attending an obstetric clinic at a gestation of 10–14 + 6 weeks from March 7, 2014, to September 7, 2016 (Accuvix V20 Prestige, Medison with 4–8 MHz volumetric transducer or EPIQ 7, Philips with X6–1 matrix transducer). The following fetal measurements were taken prospectively: crown-rump length (CRL), biparietal diameter (BPD), head circumference (HC), abdominal circumference (AC), femur length (FL), and foot length (FT). Only pregnancies with normal outcomes were included in the analysis and excluded if the entire foot could not be clearly seen during the ultrasound examination. The fetal foot length was measured from the most posterior point of the foot in its long axis to the tip of the first or the second toe whichever was longer (**Figure 1**). The estimated gestational age in weeks (GA) was calculated either from the last normal menstrual period (LMP) or from the first trimester dating scan if there was a discrepancy of more than a week [14]. This was a retrospective analysis involving minimal risk, conforming to the standards established by the NHMRC not requiring ethical review; ethics approval was therefore not sought within the institution [20].

Results for 35 ultrasound scans were analyzed with SPSS statistical package version 20 (SPSS Inc., Chicago, IL, USA). A two-sided probability (p) value of <0.05 was considered statistically significant. The regression models for the fetal measurements were obtained and would be presented in the relevant sections.

DOI: http://dx.doi.org/10.5772/intechopen.82746

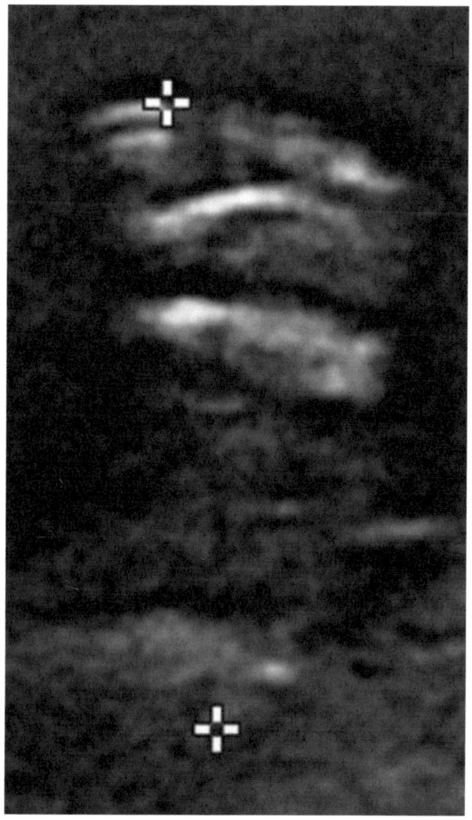

Figure 1.
Fetal foot on first trimester ultrasound scan.

3. Results

3.1 Demographic characteristics

The mean age, gravidity, and parity were 32.0 years, 2.3, and 0.7, respectively (**Table 1**). A total of 32 out of the 35 women were Asians (91.4%) and 3 were Caucasians (8.6%).

3.2 Comparison of the correlation between FT, CRL, and GA

The correlation of foot length, crown-rump length, and the gestational age assessed by date are shown in **Figures 2–4** and tabulated in **Table 2**. FT, CRL, and GA all showed positive correlation with one another in a linear fashion ($p < 0.001$)

	Mean ± S.D.	Range
Age (years)	32.0 ± 4.6	21–44
Gravidity	2.3 ± 1.5	1–8
Parity	0.7 ± 0.7	0–3

SD, standard deviation.

Table 1.
The demographic date of the pregnant women included in the study.

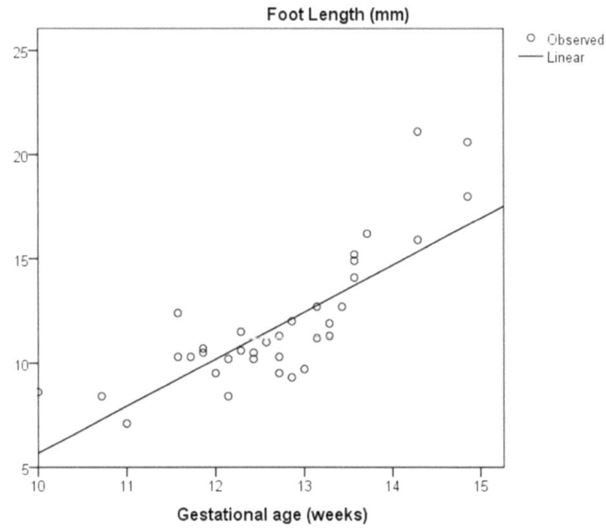

Figure 2.
The graph of fetal foot length against gestational age assessed by date. FT = GA × 2.472−19.44. R^2 = 0.675, p < 0.001. FT, foot length (mm); GA, gestational age assessed by date (weeks); R^2, coefficient of determination of regression; p, probability.

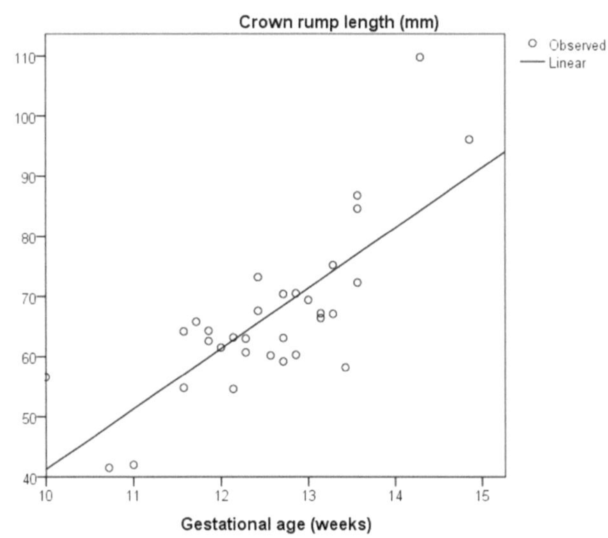

Figure 3.
The graph of fetal crown-rump length against gestational age assessed by date. CRL = GA × 10.464−64.682. R^2 = 0.608, p < 0.001. CRL, crown-rump length (mm); GA, gestational age assessed by date (weeks); R^2, coefficient of determination of regression; p, probability.

(**Figures 2–4**). The coefficient of determination of regression (R^2) was the highest between FT and CRL (0.804), lower between FL and GA (0.675), and the lowest between CRL and GA (0.608) (**Table 2**).

3.3 Comparison of the correlation of BPD, HC, AC, and FL to FT, CRL, and GA

The correlation of BPD, HC, AC, and FL with FT, CRL, and GA is shown in **Figures 5–7, 8–10, 11–13,** and **14–16**, respectively, and summarized in **Table 3**. Correlation in a linear fashion is seen for all ($p < 0.001$). Overall, the correlation

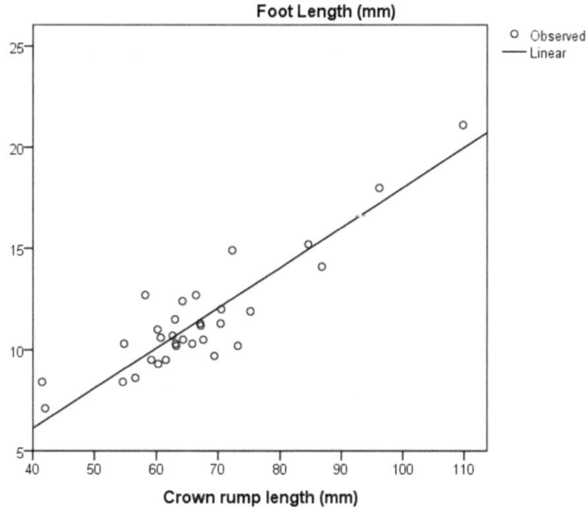

Figure 4.
The graph of fetal foot length against crown-rump length. FT = CRL × 0.187–1.074. R^2 = 0.804, p < 0.001. FT, foot length (mm); CRL, crown-rump length (mm); R^2, coefficient of determination of regression; p, probability.

Parameters	FT		CRL		GA	
	R^2	$p^{\dagger}$	R^2	$p^{\dagger}$	R^2	$p^{\dagger}$
FT	–	–	0.804	<0.001*	0.675	<0.001*
CRL	0.804	<0.001*	–	–	0.608	<0.001*
GA	0.675	<0.001*	0.608	<0.001*	–	–

*FT, foot length (mm); CRL, crown rump length (mm); GA, gestational age assessed by date (weeks); R^2, coefficient of determination of linear regression; p, probability; †, ANOVA; *, statistically significant.*

Table 2.
The correlation between fetal foot length, crown-rump length, and gestational age assessed by date.

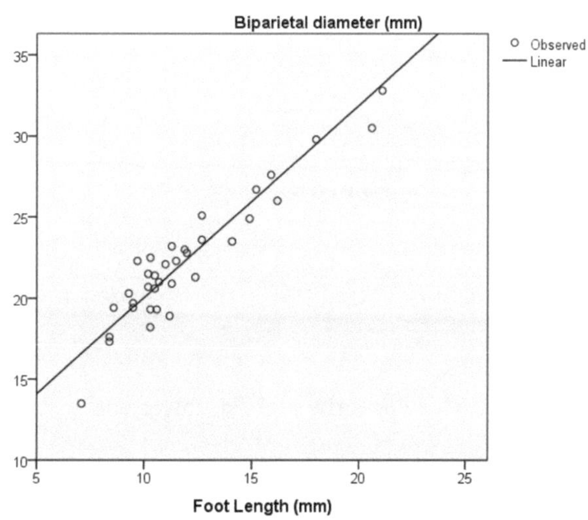

Figure 5.
The correlation of fetal biparietal diameter with foot length. BPD = FT × 1.131 + 8.748. R^2 = 0.884, p < 0.001. BPD, biparietal diameter (mm); FT, foot length (mm); R^2, coefficient of determination of regression; p, probability.

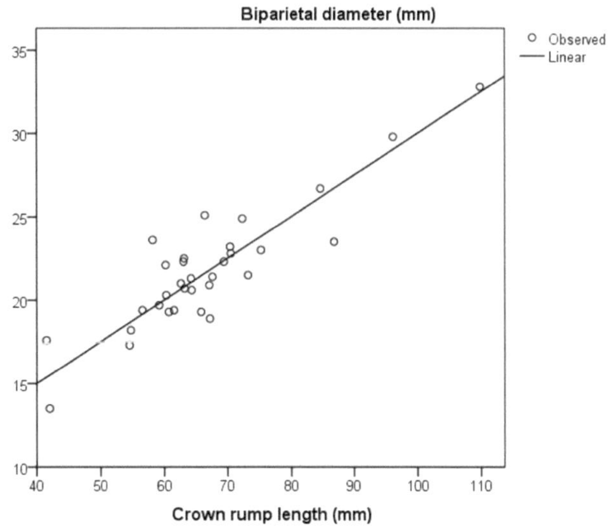

Figure 6.
The correlation of fetal biparietal diameter with crown-rump length. BPD = CRL × 0.239 + 5.78. R^2 = 0.793, $p < 0.001$. BPD, biparietal diameter (mm); CRL, crown-rump length (mm); R^2, coefficient of determination of regression; p, probability.

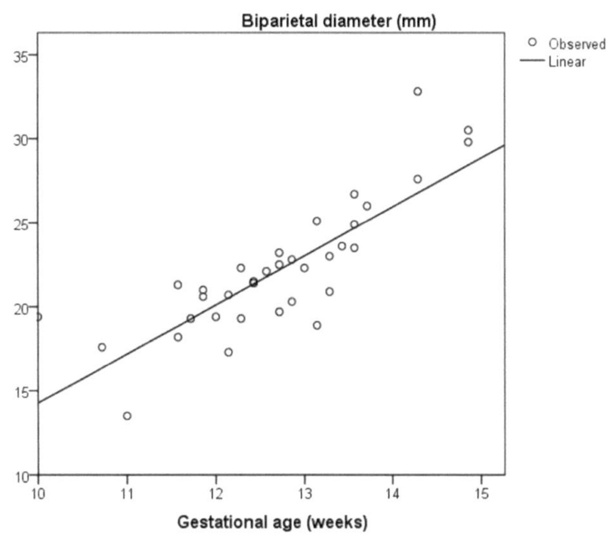

Figure 7.
The correlation of fetal biparietal diameter with gestational age assessed by date. BPD = GA × 3.01–15.967. R^2 = 0.693, $p < 0.001$. BPD, biparietal diameter (mm); GA, gestational age assessed by date (weeks); R^2, coefficient of determination of regression; p, probability.

of BPD, HC, AC, and FL with FT was the highest, lower with CRL, and the lowest with GA (**Table 3**).

3.4 Comparison of combination of fetal parameters

The correlation of combinations of fetal parameters to FT, CRL, and GA is shown in **Table 4**. The highest correlation was seen between the combination of [BPD,

HC, AC, and FL] and FT ($R^2 = 0.881$, $p < 0.001$), followed by correlation to CRL ($R^2 = 0.795$, $p < 0.001$), and the least with GA ($R^2 = 0.685$, $p < 0.001$). The addition of CRL to the combination yielded a lower R^2 value of 0.859. However, the correlation of the combination, with or without FT, to CRL yielded the same R^2 of 0.795 ($p < 0.001$).

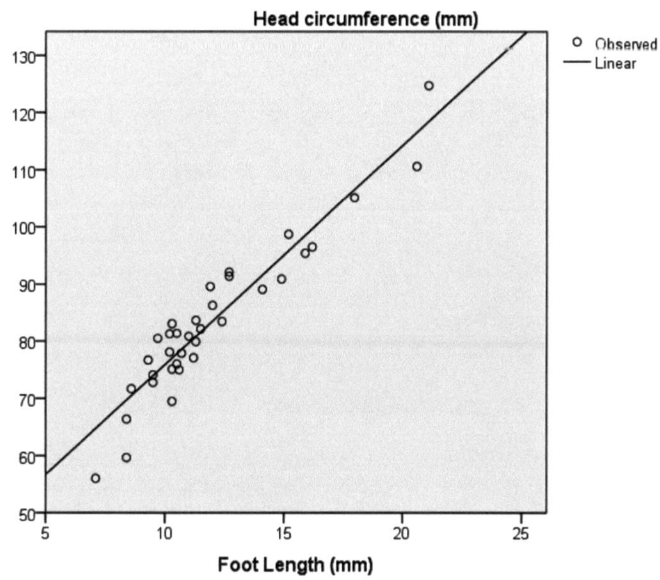

Figure 8.
The correlation of fetal head circumference with foot length. HC = FT × 3.932 + 36.257. $R^2 = 0.897$, $p < 0.001$. HC, head circumference (mm); FT, foot length (mm); R^2, coefficient of determination of regression; p, probability.

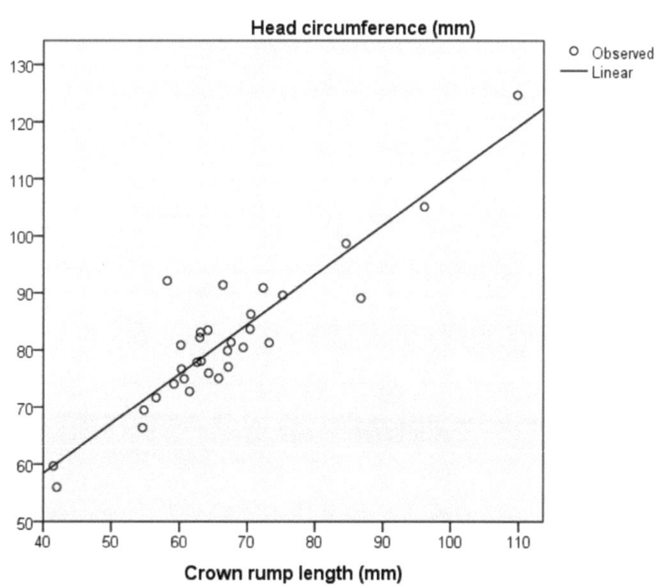

Figure 9.
The correlation of fetal head circumference with crown-rump length. HC = CRL × 0.869 + 23.646. $R^2 = 0.834$, $p < 0.001$. BPD, biparietal diameter (mm); CRL, crown-rump length (mm); R^2, coefficient of determination of regression; p, probability.

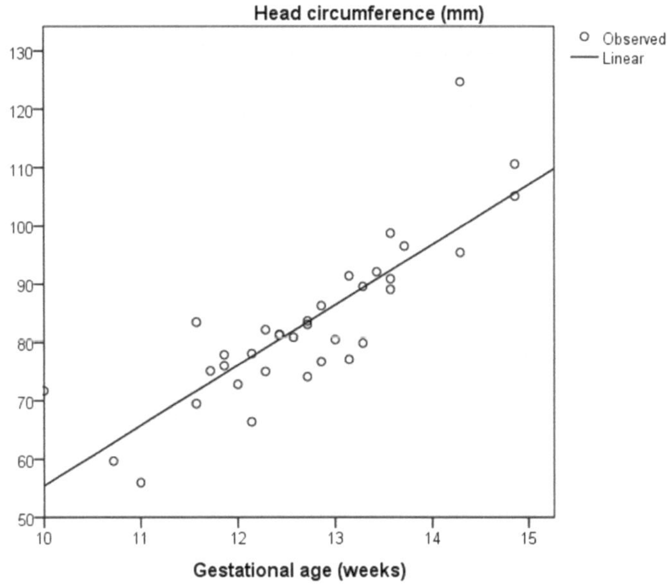

Figure 10.
The correlation of fetal head circumference with gestational age assessed by date. HC = GA × 10.488−49.951. R^2 = 0.706, p < 0.001. HC, head circumference (mm); GA, gestational age assessed by date (weeks); R^2, coefficient of determination of regression; p, probability.

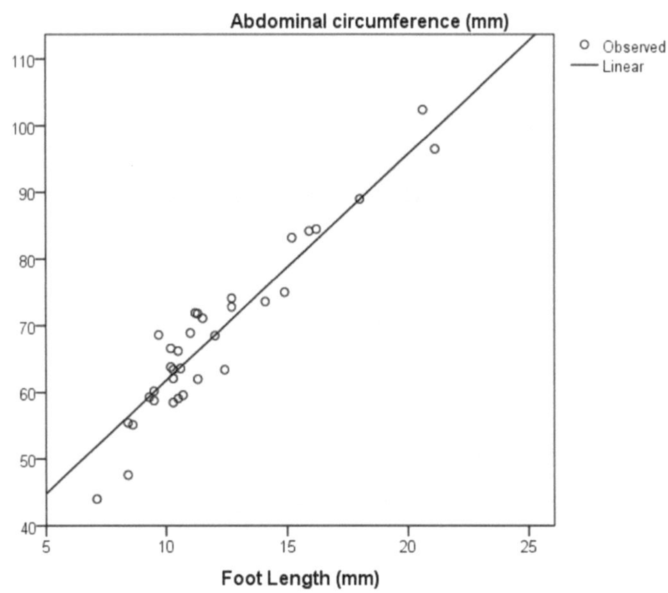

Figure 11.
The correlation of fetal abdominal circumference with foot length. AC = FT × 3.639 + 24.905. R^2 = 0.903, p < 0.001. HC, head circumference (mm); FT, foot length (mm); R^2, coefficient of determination of regression; p, probability.

The combination, in comparison to FT or CRL alone, gave a higher correlation to GA (compare to **Table 2**). However, the correlation of the combination of [BPD, HC, AC, and FL] or FT alone to CRL yielded a similar R^2 (0.795 vs. 0.804, compare **Table 4** to **Table 2**).

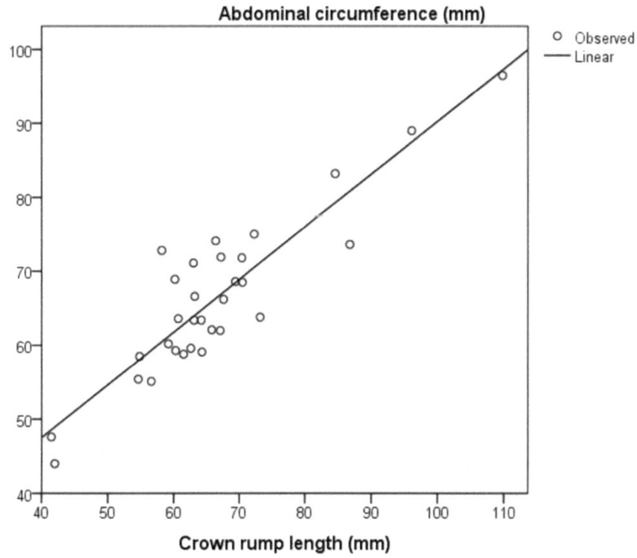

Figure 12.
The correlation of fetal abdominal circumference with crown-rump length. AC = CRL × 0.717 + 18.686. R^2 = 0.811, p < 0.001. AC, abdominal circumference (mm); CRL, crown-rump length (mm); R^2, coefficient of determination of regression; p, probability.

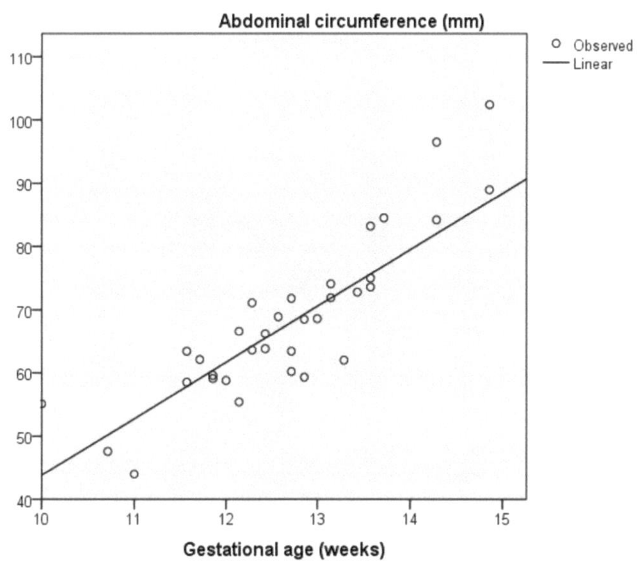

Figure 13.
The correlation of fetal abdominal circumference with gestational age assessed by date. AC = GA × 10.16–60.453. R^2 = 0.772, p < 0.001. AC, abdominal circumference (mm); GA, gestational age assessed by date (weeks); R^2, coefficient of determination of regression; p, probability.

3.5 Ratios of fetal parameters

The ratios of fetal parameters FL/FT and FL/AC to FT, CRL, GA, BPD, and HC are shown in **Figures 17–21** and **22–26**, respectively. The correlation followed an inverse relationship, and the R^2 was higher with HC or BPD or CRL or FT than GA in general (**Table 5**).

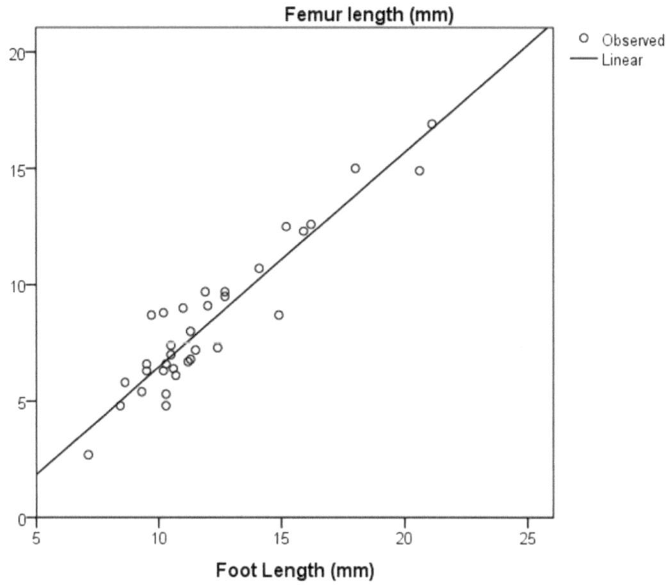

Figure 14.
The correlation of fetal femur length with foot length. FL = FT × 0.922−2.707. R^2 = 0.878, p < 0.001. FL, femur length (mm); FT, foot length (mm); R^2, coefficient of determination of regression; p, probability.

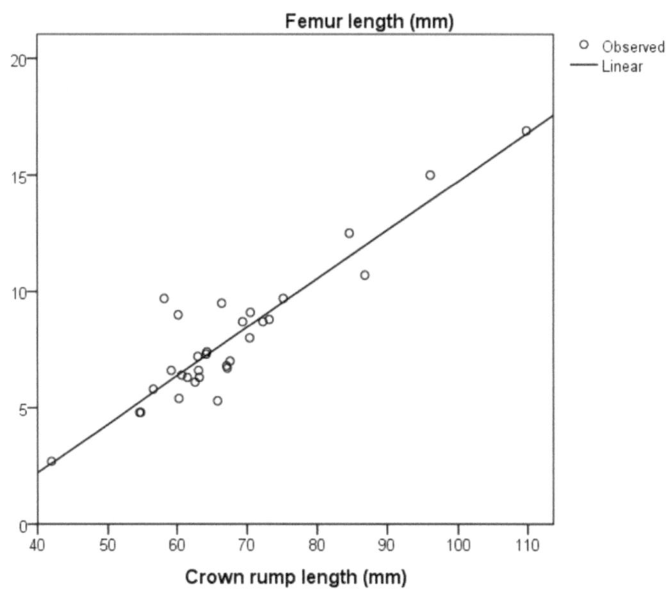

Figure 15.
The correlation of fetal femur length with crown-rump length. FL = CRL × 0.209−6.159. R^2 = 0.843, p < 0.001. FL, femur length (mm); CRL, crown-rump length (mm); R^2, coefficient of determination of regression; p, probability.

3.6 Intra- and inter-observer correlation

The Pearson coefficient for intra-observer correlation was 0.992 (p < 0.001) and for inter-observer correlation was 0.990 (p < 0.001) in the measurement of fetal foot length.

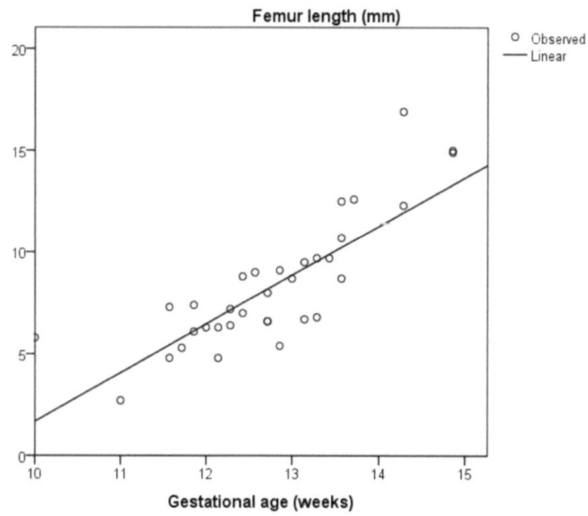

Figure 16.
The correlation of fetal femur length with gestational age assessed by date. FL = GA × 2.56−24.255. R^2 = 0.698, p < 0.001. FL, femur length (mm); GA, gestational age assessed by date (weeks); R^2, coefficient of determination of regression; p, probability.

	FT		CRL		GA	
	R^2	p†	R^2	p†	R^2	p†
BPD	0.884	<0.001*	0.793	<0.001*	0.693	<0.001*
HC	0.897	<0.001*	0.834	<0.001*	0.706	<0.001*
AC	0.903	<0.001*	0.811	<0.001*	0.772	<0.001*
FL	0.878	<0.001*	0.843	<0.001*	0.698	<0.001*
FT	–	–	0.804	<0.001*	0.675	<0.001*
CRL	0.804	<0.001*	–	–	0.608	<0.001*

*FT, foot length (mm); CRL, crown rump length (mm); GA, gestational age assessed by date (weeks); BPD, biparietal diameter (mm), HC, head circumference (mm); AC, abdominal circumference; FL, femur length (mm); R^2, coefficient of determination of regression; p, probability; †, ANOVA; *, statistically significant.*

Table 3.
The correlation of fetal biparietal diameter, head circumference, abdominal circumference, and femur length to foot length, crown-rump length, and gestational age assessed by date.

	FT		CRL		GA	
	R^2	p†	R^2	p†	R^2	p†
BPD, HC, AC, FL, FT, CRL	–	–	–	–	0.560	<0.001*
BPD, HC, AC, FL, CRL	0.859	<0.001*	–	–	0.601	<0.001*
BPD, HC, AC, FL, FT	–	–	0.795	<0.001*	0.685	<0.001*
BPD, HC, AC, FL	0.881	<0.001*	0.795	<0.001*	0.685	<0.001*

*BPD, biparietal diameter (mm); HC, head circumference (mm); AC, abdominal circumference (mm); FL, femur length (mm): FT, fetal foot length (mm); CRL, crown rump length (mm); R^2, coefficient of correlation of regression; p, probability; †, ANOVA; *, statistically significant.*

Table 4.
The correlation of multiple fetal parameters to foot length, crown-rump length, and gestational age.

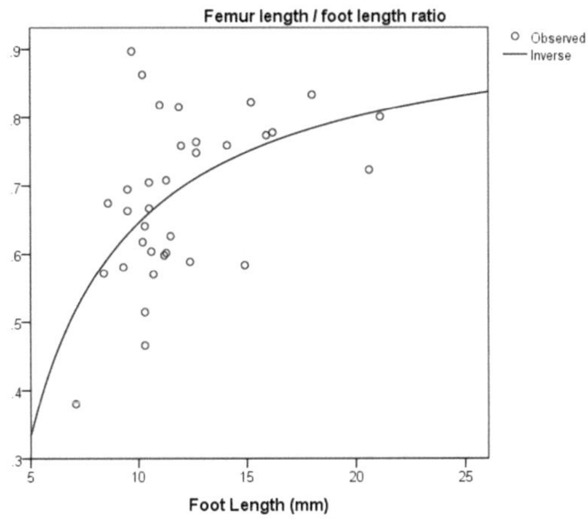

Figure 17.
The correlation of fetal femur length/foot length ratio to foot length. $R^2 = 0.283$, $p = 0.001$. R^2, coefficient of determination of regression; p, probability.

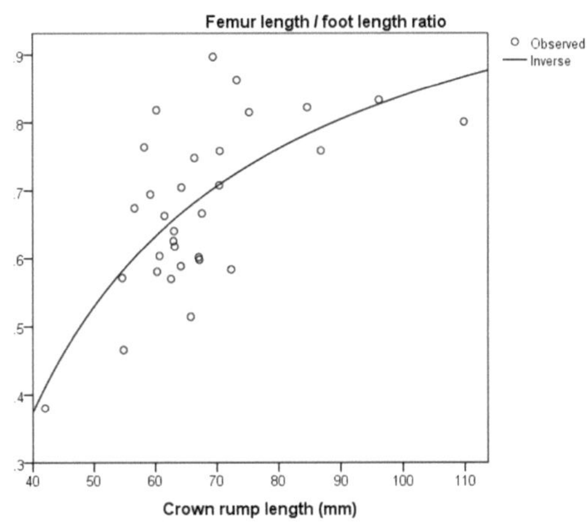

Figure 18.
The correlation of fetal femur length/foot length ratio to crown-rump length. $R^2 = 0.458$, $p < 0.001$. R^2, coefficient of determination of regression; p, probability.

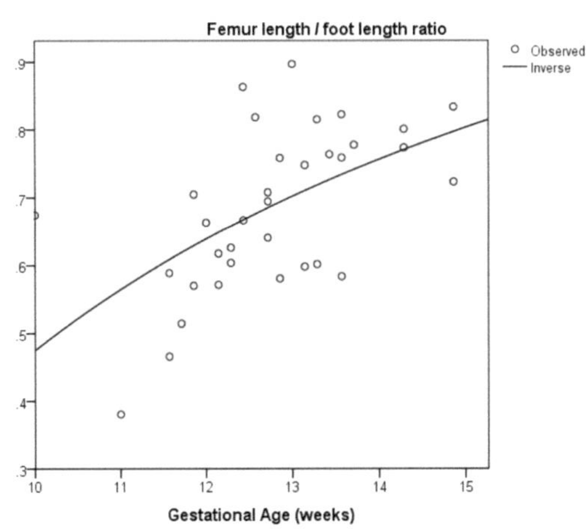

Figure 19.
The correlation of fetal femur length/foot length ratio to gestational age assessed by date. $R^2 = 0.309$, $p = 0.001$. R^2, coefficient of determination of regression; p, probability.

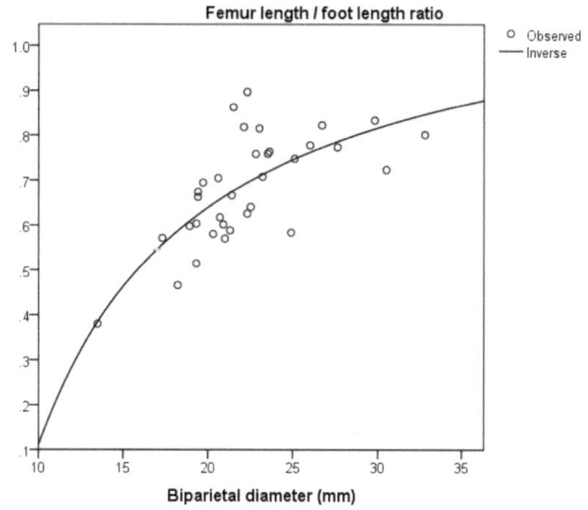

Figure 20.
The correlation of fetal femur length/foot length ratio to biparietal diameter. $R^2 = 0.522$, $p < 0.001$.
R^2, coefficient of determination of regression; p, probability.

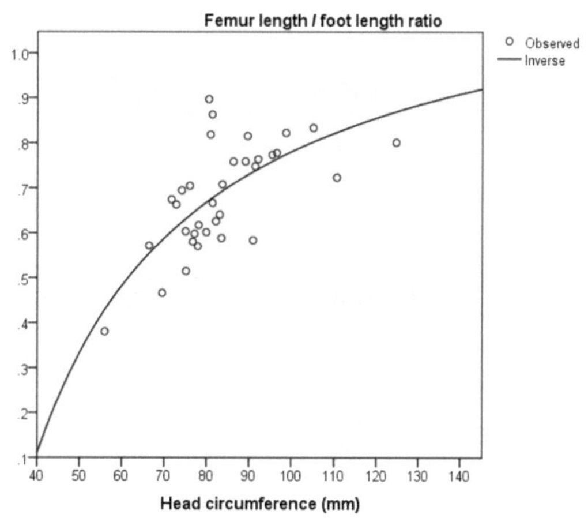

Figure 21.
The correlation of fetal femur length/foot length ratio to head circumference. $R^2 = 0.477$, $p < 0.001$.
R^2, coefficient of determination of regression; p, probability.

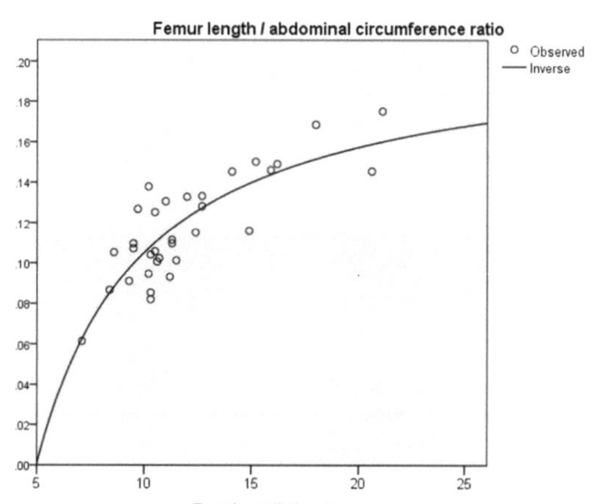

Figure 22.
The correlation of fetal femur length/abdominal circumference ratio to foot length. $R^2 = 0.684$, $p < 0.001$.
R^2, coefficient of determination of regression; p, probability.

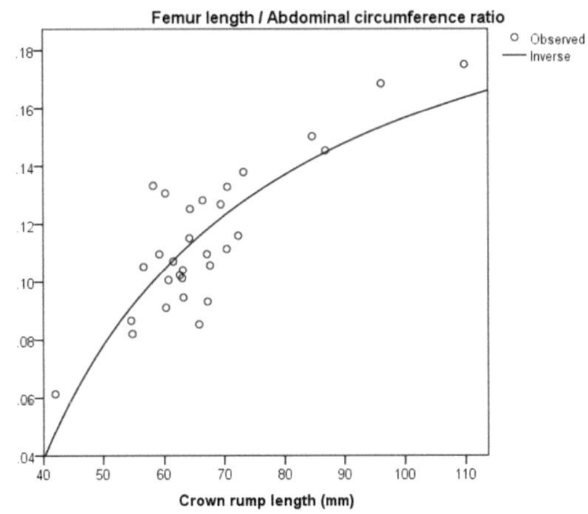

Figure 23.
The correlation of fetal femur length/abdominal circumference ratio to crown-rump length. $R^2 = 0.686$, $p < 0.001$. R^2, *coefficient of determination of regression; p, probability.*

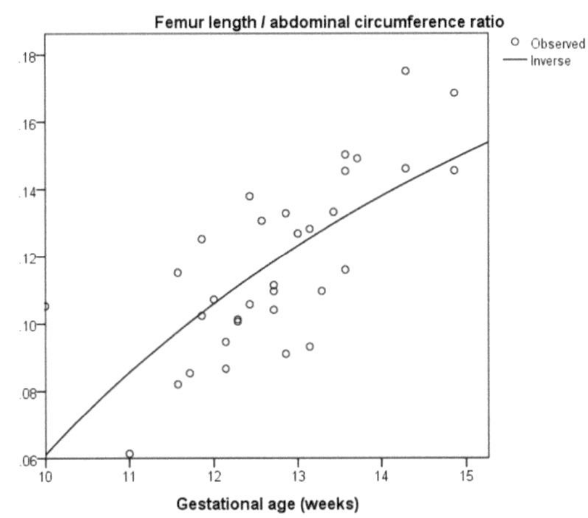

Figure 24.
The correlation of fetal femur length/abdominal circumference ratio to gestational age assessed by date. $R^2 = 0.495$, $p < 0.001$. R^2, *coefficient of determination of regression; p, probability.*

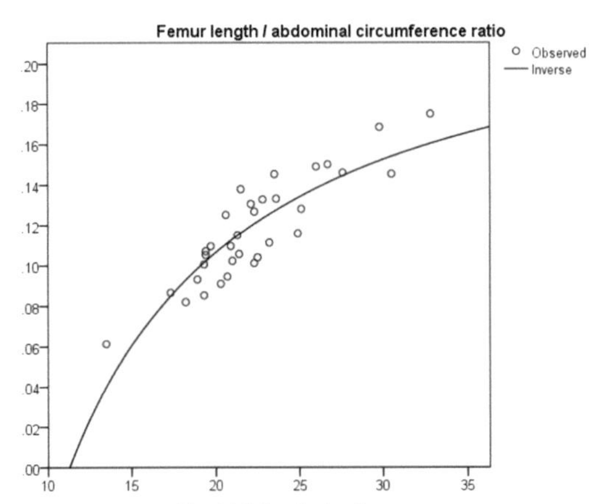

Figure 25.
The correlation of fetal femur length/abdominal circumference ratio to biparietal diameter. $R^2 = 0.765$, $p < 0.001$. R^2, *coefficient of determination of regression; p, probability.*

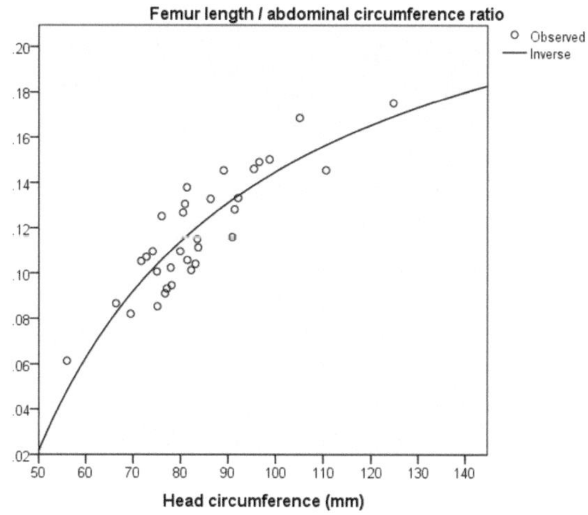

Figure 26.
The correlation of fetal femur length/abdominal circumference ratio to head circumference. R^2 = 0.773, $p < 0.001$. R^2, coefficient of determination of regression; p, probability.

	FL/AC		FL/FT	
	R^2	$p^{\dagger}$	R^2	$p^{\dagger}$
FT	0.684	<0.001*	0.283	0.001*
CRL	0.686	<0.001*	0.458	<0.001*
GA	0.495	<0.001*	0.309	0.001*
BPD	0.765	<0.001*	0.522	<0.001*
HC	0.773	<0.001*	0.477	<0.001*

*FL, femur length (mm); AC, abdominal circumference (mm); FT, foot length (mm); CRL, crown rump length (mm); GA, gestational age assessed by date (weeks); BPD, biparietal diameter (mm); HC, head circumference (mm); R^2, coefficient of determination of regression; p, probability; †, ANOVA; *, statistically significant.*

Table 5.
The correlation of foot length/abdominal circumference ratio to foot length, crown-rump length, and gestational age assessed by date, biparietal diameter, and abdominal circumference in a reverse relationship.

4. Discussion

An accurate estimation of fetal gestational age in early pregnancy is important for the assessment of the due date [14, 15] and fetal growth [21], the assignment of risk scores for the pregnancy [22], the prediction of fetal abnormality [23], and in the management of twin pregnancies [24]. CRL has been recommended as the standard parameter for assessment of fetal gestational age in the first trimester [14]. It was deduced that CRL gave a better estimation of fetal gestational age than the dates by the observation that it gave a better estimation of the date of delivery [14]. However, it is known that the measurement of CRL could be affected by the fetal posture. Variations in the estimation of fetal gestational age by a few days could be observed for the same gestation with different reference charts derived for CRL [4, 13, 25–28]. Since fetal foot length has been established as an accurate estimate for gestational age [3], it could be used as a proxy for the later. In this study, it could be seen that CRL correlates better with FT than GA. It can therefore be concluded that CRL is a better estimate of fetal gestational age than the date (**Table 2**), consistent with the previous observations [15]. However, in comparison to FT in the correlation to the other fetal parameters such as BPD, HC, AC, and FL, CRL performs less well in this study. The addition of CRL to the combination also lowers the R^2 (**Table 4**). Therefore, the use of the combination of BPD, HC, AC, and FL could well be applied from 10 to beyond 14 weeks for the estimation of fetal gestational age rather than using CRL below 14 weeks and the combination of BPD, HC, AC, and FL thereafter as in the current obstetrical practice [14]. Similarly when we use ratio of fetal parameters in the assessment of suspected fetal abnormalities, it may be better to use the ratio against fetal parameters such as FT, BPD, HC, or even CRL than against the gestational age by date, as long as the particular reference fetal parameter being used is not significantly affected by the abnormality in question (**Table 5**) [23, 29]. Of note, these ratios may not follow a linear correlation but rather an inverse relationship and vary according to the gestational age in the first trimester as alluded in a previous publication (**Figures 17–21, 22–26, Table 5**) [19].

The major limitation of the study is the sample size. The population studied comprised mainly of Asians, and hence there could be a question on generalizability. However, it has already been shown that ethnicity of the population is not an issue in sonographic estimation of fetal gestational age using crown-rump length [26]. Moreover, it has also been shown that less than 3.5% of the total variability of fetal skeletal growth was due to differences between populations when the mothers were adequately nourished [30].

With the advancement of ultrasound technology, small structures could be measured with high accuracy. Rather than relying on CRL, a parameter that could be markedly affected by fetal posture, it is perhaps time to review our ultrasound practice at 10–14 weeks in the first trimester.

5. Conclusion

In the sonographic assessment of fetal gestational age in the first trimester, the use of a combination of fetal parameters such as BPD, HC, AC, and FL is more accurate than CRL or GA at 10–14 weeks gestation in normal pregnancies. The use of these parameters as references for comparison may also be helpful when fetal abnormality is suspected in early pregnancy.

Acknowledgements

I would like to thank Dr. Hoi Yin Mary Tang of the Department of Obstetrics and Gynecology, The University of Hong Kong, for her great kindness in checking the data.

Conflict of interest

Nil to declare.

Author details

Hong Soo Wong
Australian Women's Ultrasound Centre, Hong Kong

*Address all correspondence to: wonghs.awuc@gmail.com

References

[1] Moore KL, Persaud V. Chapter 17: The limbs. In: The Developing Human Clinically Orientated Embryology. 7th ed. Philadelphia: Saunders; 2003. pp. 409-425

[2] Sadler TW. Chapter 12: Limbs. In: Langman's Medical Embryology. International Edition. 13th ed. Philadelphia: Wolters Kluwer; 2015. p. 163

[3] Streeter GL. Weight, sitting height, head size, foot length, and menstrual age of the human embryo. In: Contributions to Embryology. Vol. 11. Washington: Carnegie Institute; 1920. p. 143

[4] Mercer BM et al. Fetal foot length as a predictor of gestational age. American Journal of Obstetrics and Gynecology. 1987;**156**(2):350-355

[5] Platt LD et al. Fetal foot length: Relationship to menstrual age and fetal measurements in the second trimester. Obstetrics and Gynecology. 1988;**71**(4):526-531

[6] Goldstein I, Reece EA, Hobbins JC. Sonographic appearance of the fetal heel ossification centers and foot length measurements provide independent markers for gestational age estimation. American Journal of Obstetrics and Gynecology. 1988;**159**(4):923-926

[7] Kustermann A et al. Transvaginal sonography for fetal measurement in early pregnancy. British Journal of Obstetrics and Gynaecology. 1992;**99**(1):38-42

[8] Manjunata B, Nithin ND, Sameer S. Cross sectional study to determine gestational age by metrical measurements of foot length. Egyptian Journal of Forensic Sciences. 2012;**2**:11-17

[9] Croft MS et al. Application of obstetric ultrasound to determine the most suitable parameters for the aging of formalin-fixed human fetuses using manual measurements. Clinical Anatomy. 1999;**12**(2):84-93

[10] Hern WM. Correlation of fetal age and measurements between 10 and 26 weeks of gestation. Obstetrics and Gynecology. 1984;**63**(1):26-32

[11] Conway DL et al. An algorithm for the estimation of gestational age at the time of fetal death. Paediatric and Perinatal Epidemiology. 2013;**27**(2):145-157

[12] Hirst JE, Ha LT, Jeffery HE. The use of fetal foot length to determine stillborn gestational age in Vietnam. International Journal of Gynaecology and Obstetrics. 2012;**116**(1):22-25

[13] Robinson HP, Fleming JE. A critical evaluation of sonar "crown-rump length" measurements. British Journal of Obstetrics and Gynaecology. 1975;**82**:702-710

[14] American College of Obstetricians and Gynecologists. Committee Opinion No. 700: Methods for assessing the due date. Obstetrics and Gynecology. 2017;**129**:e150-e154

[15] Whitworth M, Bricker L, Mullan C. Ultrasound for fetal assessment in early pregnancy. Cochrane Database of Systematic Reviews. 14 Jul 2015;(7)

[16] Wong HS. A comparison of the fetal measurements for sonographic estimation of gestational age at 10 to 14 completed weeks. Indian Journal of Applied Research. 2017;7(12):647-650

[17] Khalil A, Pajkrt E, Chitty LS. Early prenatal diagnosis of skeletal anomalies. Prenatal Diagnosis. 2011;**31**(1):115-124

[18] Schramm T et al. Prenatal sonographic diagnosis of skeletal

dysplasias. Ultrasound in Obstetrics & Gynecology. 2009;**34**(2):160-170

[19] Wong HS. A revisit of the fetal foot length and fetal measurements in early pregnancy sonography. International Journal of Women's Health. 2017;**13**(9):199-204

[20] Australian Government National Health and Medical Research Council. National statement on ethical conduct in human research; 2007

[21] Reece EA et al. Dating through pregnancy: A measure of growing up. Obstetrical & Gynecological Survey. 1989;**44**(7):544-555

[22] Bindra R et al. One stop clinic for assessment of risk for trisomy 21 at 11-14 weeks: A prospective study of 15030 pregnancies. Ultrasound in Obstetrics & Gynecology. 2002;**20**:219-225

[23] Bernard JP et al. Combined screening for open spina bifida at 11-13 weeks using fetal biparietal diameter and maternal serum markers. American Journal of Obstetrics and Gynecology. 2013;**209**(3):223.e1-223.e5

[24] El Kateb A et al. First-trimester ultrasound examination and the outcome of monochorionic twin pregnancies. Prenatal Diagnosis. 2007;**27**(10):922-925

[25] McLennan AC, Schluter PJ. Construction of modern Australian first trimester ultrasound dating and growth charts. Journal of Medical Imaging and Radiation Oncology. 2008;**52**:471-479

[26] Papageorghiou AT et al. International standards for early fetal size and pregnancy dating based on ultrasound measurement of crown-rump in the first trimester of pregnancy. Ultrasound in Obstetrics & Gynecology. 2014;**44**:641-648

[27] Napolitano R et al. Pregnancy dating by fetal crown-rump length: A systematic review of charts. BJOG. 2014;**121**(5):556-565

[28] Pexters A et al. New crown-rump length curve based on over 3500 pregnancies. Ultrasound in Obstetrics & Gynecology. 2010;**35**:650-655

[29] Khalil A et al. Biparietal diameter at 11-13 weeks' gestation in fetuses with open spina bifida. Ultrasound in Obstetrics & Gynecology. 2013;**42**(4):409-415

[30] Papageorghiou AT et al. The INTERGROWTH-21st fetal growth standards: Toward the global integration of pregnancy and pediatric care. American Journal of Obstetrics and Gynecology. 2018;**218**(2S):S630-S640

Chapter 4

Undernutrition during Pregnancy

Hoang Anh Nguyen

Abstract

Experience in being pregnant is exciting but is very challenging. The term "undernutrition," as used in this chapter, focuses more on inadequate intake of energy and nutrients to meet the desired outcome of a healthy mother and her baby. Evidence shows that women with undernutrition before and during pregnancy have increased risk of metabolic disorders (i.e., gestational diabetes mellitus) and are at increased risk of complications during labor and birth. To date, nutritional therapies promoting healthier pregnancies fall into the following two major categories: (1) management of gestational weight gain and (2) the prevention or treatment of nutrient deficiencies related to pregnancy. A literature search on PubMed, the Cochrane library, Google scholar, and Cumulative Index of Nursing and Allied Health Literature was conducted to identify the relevant nutritional therapies. As a result, this chapter will analyze and discuss gestational weight gain and its effect on the health of women and her baby. The chapter briefly proposes evidence-based nutritional therapy for gestational diabetes as well as gestational common nutrient imbalance, such as vitamin D, folic acid, and omega-3 docosahexaenoic acid deficiency. The recommendations, in this chapter, would be a partial answer for these problems in Asia.

Keywords: gestational diabetes mellitus, gestational weight gain, folate deficiency, vitamin D deficiency, omega-3 docosahexaenoic acid, pregnancy outcomes

1. Introduction

The association between inadequate intake of energy and nutrients before and during pregnancy and severe maternal outcomes has been well documented in the observational studies. It is crucial for women to be fully aware of nutrition requirements without waiting until getting a positive pregnancy test result. The reason for this is that there are major changes associated with metabolism and physiology to support embryo development in the mother. The mother's diet is the only source of nutrition for her baby. Maternal undernutrition may affect the developing baby. Weight gain is a part of healthy pregnancy, but the recommendation for an optimal gestational weight gain is still controversial, especially in Asian countries. Moreover, some observational studies have shown that gestational diabetes and nutrient deficiencies during pregnancy may need to be considered differently for an individual's prenatal body mass index (BMI). Thus, in this chapter, an attempt was made to address these issues. Moreover, the role of personalized nutritional counseling, as discussed in each issue, needs to be understood carefully.

IntechOpen

2. Gestational weight gain

Getting pregnant leads to significant changes of weight in the body of women. It is normal for women to put on more weight in the last two trimesters than the first trimester as it supports the growth of fetus, the placental development, and amniotic fluid as time goes. However, putting on weight very quick per week (i.e., 0.5–1 kg in a week) is strongly associated with a life-threatening condition, such as preeclampsia [1, 2], so it is worth to notice healthcare professionals about abnormal weight gain. A woman with prepregnancy overweight and obesity should take a plan of gestational weight gain GWG into account during prenatal visits. A cohort study of 3539 women with a follow-up period of 17 years demonstrated that overweight women (BMI > 25) at the beginning of pregnancy had an increased risk of diabetes, cardiac disease, or endocrine diseases later in their life [1]. Moreover, excessive or inadequate weight-gain levels during pregnancy can affect small or large gestational age, an increased risk of cesarean delivery, and other adverse pregnancy outcomes, including gestational diabetes mellitus and preeclampsia [1–4].

The Worth Health Organization definition of body mass index (BMI) is "a person's weight in kilograms divided by the square of the person's height in meters (kg/m^2)." For instance, a pregnant woman who weighs 50 kg and her height is 1.6 m will have a BMI of 19.5. BMI has been well recognized as an effective measurement to identify overweight and subsequent health risks in an individual. The increasing level of BMI from overweight to extreme obese is thought to accompany the increasing risk of health problems (Canadian Health Guideline 2004). The American Institute of Medicine (IOM) recommended the ideal amount of weight gained during pregnancy based on WHO-BMI ranges from underweight to obesity, but not all obesity classes were addressed (**Table 1**). The origin of the IOM recommendations about gestational weight gain (GWG) came primarily from the American population-based studies despite its popular applicability to European and Asian countries. In the Asian population-based studies reviewed, the recommendations of the IOM concerning gestational weight gain (GWG) have limited applicability for Asian women to get their desired GWG. The accumulated evidence on noncommunicable diseases demonstrated that Asian adults get more body fat and have greater risks of diabetes and cardiovascular diseases at their lower BMI in comparison with non-Asian population. Thus, Asian regional BMI cutoff points [6] developed by the panel of WHO consultation minimize these risks (**Table 2**). A large meta-analysis study with more than 300,000 Asian women confirmed that the IOM recommendations about GWG can be applicable in Asian countries when using regional BMI cutoff points for overweight or obese [7]. The evidence was not attempted to define a GWS guideline for all Asian women as the data of this study were based primarily on East Asian countries, such as China, Taiwan, Korea, and Japan. Moreover, Korean and Taiwanese women tend to gain more weight during pregnancy than other Asian women [8]. This requires more comparative studies in Asia. However, its strength confirmed that the guideline for GWG may need to be considered differently for Asian women. To date, a global consensus regarding a desired GWG is still understudied.

Recommendations	Underweight	Normal weight	Overweight	Obese
Prenatal BMI (kg/m^2)	<18.5	18.5–24.9	25.0–29.9	≥30
Total weight gain range (kg)	12.5–18	11.5–16	7–11.5	5–9

Table 1.
Recommended weight gain during pregnancy based on the 2009 Institute of Medicine (IOM) guideline [5].

	Asian BMI cutoff points (kg/m^2)	Total weight gain range (kg)*
Underweight	<18.5	12.5–18
Normal weight	18.5–22.9	11.5–16
Overweight	23–27.5	7–11.5
Obese	27.6–29.9 ≥30	7–11.5 5–9

**These recommendations suggested by the author should only be used as a reference for public health strategists, nutritional practitioners, or healthcare professionals in Asia. These recommendations were based on ideas in a large meta-analysis study [7]; thus, they are not considered as a completed guideline.*

Table 2.
The proposed gestational weight gain recommendation based on Asian regional BMI cutoff points [6].

An excessive amount of weight gained during pregnancy could be predictive of weight retention at 6 months postpartum [2] and of an increased risk of weight management challenges later in life [3, 4]. A meta-analytic study of over 65,000 women by Nehring et al. demonstrated that women with GWG above the IOM recommendations were likely to have an additional gain of 3 kg at 3 years and of 4.7 kg at 15 years after pregnancy, compared to those with GWG within the recommendations [3].

2.1 Brief nutrition recommendations for gestational weight gain

Transitions to a new weight gain during a pregnancy may need to meet additional calories every day. According to the IOM expert panel's recommendation on macronutrients for pregnant women with normal BMI, an estimation of additional 0, 340, and 452 kcal for the first, second, and third trimester, respectively [9, 10] was recommended. Moreover, additional calories should also be personalized to an individual's prenatal BMI [10].

- If prenatal BMI is less than 18.5 kg/m^2, the mother needs to begin an additional 150 kcal per day for her first 3 months, and continuously add 50 and 150 kcal for her second and third trimester, respectively. They can benefit from protein supplements [10].

- If women are overweight or obese, they do not need to add calories in their first trimester. In two last trimesters, they need to add between 450 and 500 kcal per day to meet their gestational weight gain. Prenatal overweight or obesity is strongly associated with an increased risk of pregnancy complications as well as postpartum weight retention. They may need supports to lose weight effectively during prenatal visits. Evidence has shown that overweight or obese women who reduced at least 3 BMI units before conception can lower the chance of developing gestational diabetes by two-fold [10, 11].

- For multiple pregnancy, woman with normal BMI should consume about 40–45 kcal/kg/day while an estimated 30–35 and 42–50 kcal/kg/day have been advised for overweight and underweight BMI, respectively [12–14].

Adding small meals or one or two extra snacks during the day may facilitate these targets. There is no need to stick on high-energy density diets, but, a balanced diet with nutrient-dense foods has the benefit of providing a range of vitamins and minerals.

3. Management of gestational diabetes mellitus during pregnancy

Gestational diabetes mellitus (GDM) is one of the common pregnancy complications related to diet. Pregnancy is related with a biological reduction of insulin sensitivity by about 60% [15], which supports fetus development by an increase of glucose into the placenta. Some women were present with elevated blood glucose levels during their pregnancy although no diabetes was diagnosed before their pregnancy. The excessive blood glucose level can cause hyperglycemia which will develop gestational diabetes mellitus. Fortunately, the well-managed blood glucose levels typically turn normal after delivery. GDM globally happens in about 3–28% of pregnant women. The prevalence of GDM in European countries is about 5.4%, while 10.1% GDM occurs in Eastern and Southeastern Asian countries, except in Indonesia, the Philippines, Myanmar, Cambodia, and Laos [16]. Among the latter, Vietnam and Singapore have the greatest prevalence of GDM (about 20%). The prevalence of diabetes during a pregnancy has been increasing markedly in Africa and Asia [16]. It is closely associated with the increase of obesity and sedentary lifestyle. It is the most common medical complication during a pregnancy. Women with a healthy weight can be affected. This is likely due to participation of pregnancy-related hormones, such as human placental lactogen (HPL). A 30-fold increase of HPL by the 20th week of gestation causes improperly elevated blood sugar levels, which contributes to the developing GDM between the second and the third trimester [17, 18]. However, women who enter into pregnancy overweight or obese are at a markedly increased risk of developing GDM. The increased release of pro-inflammatory cytokines and adiponectin was associated with an accumulation of adipose tissues, particularly with central obesity [19–21]. These releases contribute to a severe GDM, including increased glucose blood levels [22], endoplasmic reticulum stress [23], and increased insulin resistance [21, 24]. Women, diagnosed with a lower adiponectin concentration at their early trimester, are likely to develop an increased insulin resistance and GDM later in their semesters [25].

Several adverse outcomes are associated with diabetes during a pregnancy: mothers with the untreated GDM have a higher risk of hypertension, preeclampsia, cesarean delivery, and labor complications; their babies are at increased risk of macrosomia, large for gestational age, fetal organomegaly, shoulder dystocia, hypoglycemia, and perinatal morbidity and mortality due to the excessive glucose flux into the placenta [26, 27].

3.1 Nutritional therapy for gestational diabetes mellitus

The role of nutrition in the management of gestational diabetes mellitus is now drawing considerable attention in public because of the natural process without side effects for women and their unborn baby. Diet-based interventions in the pregnancy aim to control maternal hyperglycemia as well as to lower risks of macrosomia. The concept of these interventions is a three-step nutritional therapy (NT), including a personalized dietary counseling, appropriate energy restriction, and promotion of a balanced diet.

Some observational studies reviewed that it is beneficial for women to take three-step NT into consideration in prenatal or early pregnancy visits if they have one or more of the following contributory factors for GDM [28–30]:

1. Being overweight or obese (BMI cut offs ≥ 23 kg/m^2 for Asian population; BMI ≥ 25 kg/m^2 for non-Asian population)

2. Having GDM or abnormal glucose tolerance in previous pregnancy

3. Having diagnosed polycystic ovary syndrome (PCOS)

4. Having macrosomia in previous pregnancy (birth weight > 4 kg)

5. Having a family member with diabetes

6. Hypertension (140/90 mm Hg) [12] or recurrent hypertension

7. Secondary lifestyle

8. HDL <35 mg/dL, triglyceride >250 mg/dL

9. High risk race: Asian, Indian subcontinent, Aboriginal and Torres Strait Islander, Pacific Islander, Maori, Middle Eastern, non-white African.

3.2 A personalized counseling for GDM

Women with diagnosed gestational diabetes need to be put on a proper diet. Thus, they should seek a tailored nutritional counseling by a registered nutritional therapist. Personalized dietary counseling was associated with a well-controlled maternal hyperglycemia and a proper weight gain due to the mothers' better awareness about GDM and meal plans [31, 32]. The dietary counseling needs to be tailored for an individual; this consists of things like not only her diet and lifestyle but her expectation and barrier. For instance, the nutritional advice on a restricted diet of fast foods should also discuss about where a patient can get healthy foods and her related barriers. Moreover, understanding the effects of the dietary advice on not only an individual but also her family members has shown the significant improvement of clinical outcomes [33, 34]. This is likely due to family member's additional support.

Some meta-analysis and systematic review studies demonstrated that women with GDM had encountered the weight management, in particular overweight or obese people [32]. A majority of these cases are largely associated with their unhealthy lifestyle choices, including low physical activities, problematic portion control, and poor diet. In the context, the counseling needs to take these issues into consideration. Moreover, it is important to promote healthy food choices in the consultation. Importantly, the nutritional advice for GDM is tailored, relevant, and applicable to the patient.

3.3 Energy restriction and appropriate weight gain for GDM

Energy restriction aims to ensure that women and their babies get enough energy to develop and grow, but minimizes the reductant amount of weight gained. The influence of energy balance on dietary macronutrient intake and physical activity could be considered as a primary factor in the reduced fat composition. There is some established evidence that moderate caloric restriction can improve maternal hyperglycemia as well as reduce insulin requirement, but, there is no association between restricted caloric intake and birth weight. However, severe caloric restriction to either less than 1200 kcal per day or 50% of daily energy requirement is related to the production of ketonuria and ketonemia, which is called ketosis [35, 36]. According to the recommendations of American Diabetes Association about energy restriction, obese women with GDM can benefit from a 30–33% energy restriction or a limit of 25 kcal per kg per day, but there was no report related to GDM women with normal weight [35, 37, 38]. Some studies suggested a caloric restriction of 30–34 kcal/kg (actual weight of pregnant women) for those with normal BMI [36]. However, further interventional studies are needed to take this recommendation into action.

3.4 Promotion of a balanced diet with high fiber and low carbohydrate

The transport of glucose into the placenta depends on how accelerated the mother's postprandial blood glucose concentrations are. The excessive amount of glucose crosses the placenta, which can affect birth weight. A postprandial high blood glucose levels in GDM women is typically higher. Insulin is a metabolic hormone released from beta-cells in the pancreas, which play an essential role in the blood glucose regulation. Dietary carbohydrate is absorbed into the intestine and converted into simple glucose, which leads to a significant increase of maternal blood glucose concentrations. After a meal, GDM women found normoglycemia very challenging. They sometimes need medications to turn their blood glucose normal. One of the major purposes in the GDM nutritional management is thus to achieve normoglycemia after meal. The postprandial blood glucose level depends on the amount of glucose absorbed in the intestine and released into the bloodstream. There is some established evidence that a diet rich in fibrous carbohydrate, such as vegetables and fruits, and low in starchy and high glycemic index carbohydrate, may be helpful to reduce postprandial blood glucose as well as to change body fat composition [39, 40]. The American Diabetes Association guideline focuses on how much energy from dietary carbohydrate a GDM woman consumes [41]. The guideline demonstrated that the consumption of dietary carbohydrate among women with GDM should be limited to 40–45% of total daily energy, with a smaller percentage at breakfast than at lunch or dinner.

Glycemic index (GI) is a measurement related to the amount of carbohydrate in certain foods and its effect on a blood glucose increase after eating, a rank of values from 0 to 100. A high GI in foods (≥70) causes a sharp increase in blood glucose compared with a food with a medium (56–69) or low GI (≤55). Some established evidence recommended that the GDM women can consume low GI or complex carbohydrates, even greater than 45% of the total energy, without a quick response of increased blood glucose [42, 43]. Glycemic control can be achieved by increasing the consumption of foods with low GI, such as whole grains, green vegetables, and legumes, instead of high-GI foods like potatoes or sweet foods. Rice, a starchy food, is routinely eaten by 60% of world population, primarily in Asian countries. Approximately three-fourths of the total carbohydrate calorie requirement in Southeast Asia comes from rice [44]. Like potatoes or white breads in western countries, white rice can be a staple part of Asian meals. Unfortunately, the refined white rice may increase risk of hyperglycemia. It is a challenge for Asian women with GDM to avoid white rice due to its preferred taste or flavor, but following a low-GI diet guideline along with white rice will facilitate their glycemic control (**Table 3**). Several conventional studies demonstrated that the different types of rice have variations in GI value. For instance, among 12 types of rice commercially available in the United Kingdom, a nonblind, randomized trial indicated that rice noodles, long-grain rice, white basmati rice, and easy-cook long-grain rice were classified as low-GI foods, compared with others [45]. This is likely due to the difference in amylose composition and its effect on gelatinization [46, 47] rather

Groups	Foods
Starchy foods	Limit a cup of white rice a day. Avoid white rice or glutinous rice in breakfast or late dinner. Swap white rice for the low-GI starchy foods, such as rice noodles, brown rice, udon noodles, whole spaghetti, and sweet corn. Should be chosen preferentially
Raw Fruits	***Swap fruit juices or soft-drinks for low-GI raw fruits***, such as apple, orange, grapefruit, green grape, and banana; 1–2 servings (80–160 g) a day. ***Accepted fruit juices***: Apple and orange
Vegetables and legumes	Boiled/steamed/raw vegetables or vegetable soups from carrots, sweet potato, pumpkin, green banana and green leafy vegetables (i.e., spinach, green broccoli, or Moringa leaves); 3–4 servings (240–320 g) per day. ***Low-GI legumes***: red kidneys, soy beans, and black beans; 1–2 servings per week.
Dairy products	Natural/white yogurts; 1–2 servings a day.
Meats	About 20% of total energy with smaller proportions in red meats than oily fish and chicken.
Things to avoid	• Fast foods and animal fat or skin. • Skipping meals. • Alcohol or alcoholic drinks. • Drinking soft drinks or sugary foods between meals. • Very big meal; keeping meals medium sized and regular will prevent hyperglycemia throughout the day. Additional healthy snacks would be beneficial.

Table 3.
Recommended low-GI diet for Asian pregnancy with GDM.

than the dietary fiber content solely [46]. Rice with higher amylose composition has greater GI. The gelatinization represents the thickening of starch granules when heated in the presence of water. Thus, rice with greater gelatinization, such as glutinous rice, will have higher GI [48].

The evidence stated that the consumption of a high amount of fat, particularly with saturated fatty acids, can affect both the insulin-induced signaling pathway on cell membranes and lipid metabolism after a meal [49, 50]. Saturated fatty acids in strong relation to insulin resistance are well documented in not only epidemiological but also intervention studies [51]. Moon demonstrated that diets rich in saturates appear to impair the insulin-induced normal signaling by reducing IRS-1 expression and phosphorylated PI3K levels [52]. This results in significantly decreased transfer of glucose across the muscle cell membrane via GLUT-4, glucose transporter proteins, and the increased serum glucose. In addition, in a current study on mice with impaired Toll-like receptor-4, Zhou also demonstrated that saturated fatty acids are associated with glucose intolerance through reducing functions of nucleotide-binding oligomerization domain 1 (NOD1) in insulin-stimulated glucose uptake in adipocytes [53]. Thus, women with GDM may need to avoid saturated fats, but increase consumption of polyunsaturated fatty acids, especially fish oil [54]. A randomized double-blinded, placebo-controlled trial on fish oil supplementation and its effects on GDM demonstrated that omega-3 supplementation was associated with upgraded expression of genes related to insulin activities and inflammation among GDM women [55]. To date, taking omega-3 supplements routinely has not been recommended for the treatment of GDM due to lack of evidence. However, omega-3 supplements may need to be considered additionally for pregnant women if they find fish consumption challenging.

4. Management of vitamin D deficiency during pregnancy

Vitamin D is essential for absorption of dietary calcium and phosphate in the small intestine and for the deposition of calcium and phosphate in the mother's bones, and for her baby's as well. Moreover, maternal vitamin D was known as the only source for the unborn baby. Gestational vitamin D deficiency during pregnancy is related to infantile rickets. Moreover, the lack of vitamin D in the first trimester of pregnancy is predictable to preeclampsia and gestational diabetes mellitus [56, 57]. Maternal vitamin D is primarily synthesized under her skin while exposed to sunlight. First, due to sunlight, the 7-dehydrocholesterol under skin will be converted into cholecalciferol (vitamin D3). Then, the hydroxylation of vitamin D3 in the liver occurs to form 25(OH)D. Finally, 25(OH)D is continuously hydroxylated in the kidney to become a biologically more active form, 1,25(OH)2D. Serum 25(OH)D concentrations are clinically measured to indicate an individual's vitamin D status due to its stable half-life of 2–3 weeks. There is some established evidence that inadequate serum vitamin D concentrations at early childhood puts individuals into a higher risk of metabolic disorders later in their life, such as heart disease and diabetes as vitamin D receptors are present in almost tissues.

Those women who smoke, use sunscreen, or cover their skin with clothing increase significantly risk of vitamin D deficiency. Unfortunately, some individuals have encountered getting an adequate amount of vitamin D due to their darker skin tone. A global sunshine calendar developed by the Vitamin D Day (https://www.vitamindday.net/) suggested a practical tip for an individual to get enough vitamin D while exposed to sunlight, no matter where he or she lives.

One of the biggest concerns about getting vitamin D from sun is skin cancer due to ultraviolet (UV) radiation exposure. There was an association between less education and misconception of vitamin D from sunlight. A cross-sectional survey of 3922 participants in the United States demonstrated that individuals with a high school diploma or less had misconception of a longer sunlight exposure related to achievement of a sufficient vitamin D, which may need more studies about vitamin D-related sun exposure behaviors and risk of skin cancer [58]. In natal visits, it is important for registered nutritional practitioners to take women's vitamin D knowledge as well as their sun safety behaviors into consideration [59].

Mushroom, oily fish, egg yolks, and vitamin D fortified milk is a dietary source of vitamin D. Oral vitamin D supplementation is as available as drops or tables, which can be taken over the counter or on registered nutritional practitioner's prescription. Oral vitamin D supplementations among pregnant population have shown to improve maternal vitamin D status and lower risk of premature birth delivery. According to the guideline of the Royal College of Obstetrics and Gynecology (RCOG), a daily vitamin D supplementation of 400 units is recommended for women with singleton gestation [60]. To date, there is still no vitamin D guideline for twin or multiple pregnancies although it shares an increased risk of gestational outcomes. Some experts from the Society of Maternal Fetal Medicine suggested that women with twin gestations should consume daily vitamin D supplementations of 1000 units [61]. Oral vitamin D supplementations within the guideline, plus sunlight exposure, will not lead to symptoms of excessive vitamin D.

There is a hypothetical concern that which is better: taking vitamin D supplementation alone or in combination with calcium? The evidence from a Cochrane systematic review confirmed that the consumption of vitamin D combined with calcium is related to an increased risk of premature birth [62]. The effect and cause behind the evidence were not well documented. Thus, it is important for the registered nutritional practitioners or nutritional therapist to take measures to manage this risk when making a description of vitamin D combined with calcium for preeclampsia. It is beneficial for public to take vitamin D supplement alone over the counter within the guideline.

Women who enter into pregnancy obese are also at increased risk of nutrient deficiencies, in particular, deficiencies of vitamin D. Also in pregnant women, BMI is inversely associated with the serum concentrations of vitamin D. Obese women are at a markedly increased risk of vitamin D deficiency compared to women with BMI in the normal range, and the offsprings of obese women also have lower levels of vitamin D in their cord blood. The prevalence of vitamin D deficiency in pregnant women can be quite high in some populations, reaching, for example, one third in the USA, 35% in the UK, and 77% in Germany [63]. Vitamin D is believed to be sequestered in the adipose tissue, making it less available in obese people.

Hence, obese women have an even higher prevalence of vitamin D deficiency during pregnancy. Recently, the RCOG guidelines recommended that obese pregnant women should be taking at least 1000 units a day of vitamin D supplementation, compared with a daily vitamin D supplementation of 400 units for those women with healthy BMI [60, 64].

Women at higher risk of vitamin D deficiency, such as obesity, need to follow a maternal vitamin D assessment in prenatal, first trimester, and last trimester visits to ensure a proper vitamin D supplementation.

5. Management of folic acid deficiency during pregnancy

Folate or vitamin B9, a family member of water-soluble vitamins, plays an important role in the production of neurotransmitters and synthesis of DNA in cells, especially in early pregnancy. Folate is naturally found in dark green leafy vegetables and legumes while folic acid, a synthetic form of vitamin B9, is generally added in supplements or fortified milk or foods. Folate deficiency in pregnancy generally occurs when maternal dietary supply does not meet a suddenly increased folate requirement for the embryogenesis [65]. This requires an adequate amount of folate prior to conception and continuing throughout within next 28 days, an essential period of neural tube formation. The failure will lead to abnormal fetus development, even death. New parents are often unaware of their pregnancy as well as unprepared of an increased folate demand of this important event [65, 66].

All pregnant women need to consume a daily folate supplementation of 400 μg or 0.4 mg. Folate deficiency is strongly associated with abnormal neural tube development. Evidence has shown that the risk of neural tube defects among obese pregnant women is double that of women with normal BMI. As a result, a higher dosage of folate supplementation is recommended for pregnant women with high BMI. It is important for these women to take this raised amount of folic acid at least a month prior to conception to their first trimester. The Center for Maternal and Child Enquiry jointly with the Royal College of Obstetrics and Gynecology recommends that women with a body mass index higher than 29.9 should take a supplement on top of their diet, with 5 mg of folic acid daily [67]. In contrast, the recommended folic acid dosage for women with a healthy BMI, of course, is only 0.4 mg daily.

6. DHA in a pregnancy

Omega-3 docosahexaenoic acid (DHA; 22:6n-3) is an important component in the cell membrane, specially brain cells. It has been postulated that low maternal

DHA concentrations could be related with increased risk of postpartum depression and preterm birth. During the embryogenesis, maternal DHA levels significantly increased, which may contribute to reduce oxidative stress-induced impairment of the neurotrophic factors [68]. Omega-3 DHA is pronouncedly found in a fetus brain from the last trimester to 12 months after delivery [69, 70]. Oily fish, river eels, and wide carps are often a rich source of omega-3 essential fatty acids (FA). DHA in the diet can be obtained from river eels, wide carps, and marine-derived fatty fish, such as salmon, mackerel, anchovies, sardines, and sea trout. One of the biggest concerns about seafood consumption is risk of mercury exposure. According to the United States Environmental Protection Agency (EPA)'s fish advice, it is safe for pregnant women to consume 2 servings (6.2 ounces or 175 g) of certain cooked fish with a low average mercury concentration (≤ 0.15 μg/g) [71, 72]. Some oily fish species labeled as "the best choice to consume" are Atlantic mackerels, anchovies, herrings, haddocks, lobsters, salmon, sardine, and light tuna. However, women, who might become pregnant, should avoid or consume less than 100 g per week predatory fish species, such as bigeye tuna, swordfish, marline, shark, and orange roughy [73–75]. Alternatively, oral DHA supplementation alone of 200–300 mg was recommended for all pregnant women [72].

7. Conclusion

Based on the present work, there are three main conclusions which may help women have a healthy baby during their pregnancy. First, an increase in body weight is necessary during the last two trimesters. However, the gestational weight gain should be interpreted with some cautions related to prenatal BMI, especially overweight or underweight. Second, gestational diabetes is strongly associated with a greater risk of poor pregnancy outcomes. Once diagnosed, diet-based interventions aim to control maternal hyperglycemia. As a result, seeking a tailored nutritional counseling by a registered nutritional therapist will put on a proper diet, including the appropriate management of energy restriction and the promotion of a balanced diet with high fiber and low GI carbohydrate. Moreover, the management of blood glucose during pregnancy may benefit from avoiding saturated fats, but increasing consumption of polyunsaturated fatty acids. Last, it has clearly been shown that pregnant women may find it harder to consume enough specific nutrients, such as vitamin D, folate, and omega-3 DHA. Consuming fortified or enriched foods or oral nutrient supplementations may optimize a diet.

Author details

Hoang Anh Nguyen[1,2,3]*

1 British Association for Nutrition and Lifestyle Medicine, UK

2 Nutrition Informatics and Genomics Unit, Child Nutrition Foundation (CNF), UK

3 Nutrition Therapy, University of Worcester, Worcester, UK

*Address all correspondence to: stevenguyen.uk.hcm@gmail.com

References

[1] Moll U, Olsson H, Landin-Olsson M. Impact of pregestational weight and weight gain during pregnancy on long-term risk for diseases. PLoS One. 2017; **12**(1):e0168543. DOI: 10.1371/journal.pone.0168543

[2] Haugen M, Brantsaeter AL, Winkvist A, et al. Associations of pre-pregnancy body mass index and gestational weight gain with pregnancy outcome and postpartum weight retention. A prospective observational cohort study. BMC Pregnancy and Childbirth. 2014; **14**:201. DOI: 10.1186/1471-2393-14-201

[3] Nehring I, Schmoll S, Beyerlein A, Hauner H, von Kries R. Gestational weight gain and long-term postpartum weight retention. A meta-analysis. The American Journal of Clinical Nutrition. 2011;**94**(5):1225-1231

[4] Kirkegaard H, Stovring H, Rasmussen KM, Abrams B, Sorensen TI, Nohr EA. How do pregnancy-related weight changes and breastfeeding relate to maternal weight and BMI adjusted waist circumference 7 year after delivery? Results from a path analysis. The American Journal of Clinical Nutrition. 2014;**99**(2):312-319

[5] Institute of Medicine. Weight Gain During Pregnancy: Reexamining the Guidelines. Washington, D.C: The National Academies Press; 2009

[6] WHO Expert Consultation. Appropriate body-mass index for Asian populations and its implications for policy and intervention strategies. Lancet. 2004;**363**:157-163

[7] Goldstein RF, Abell SK, Ranasinha S, Misso ML, Boyle JA, Harrison CL, et al. Gestational weight gain across continents and ethnicity: Systematic review and meta-analysis of maternal and infant outcomes in more than one million women. BMC Medicine. 2018; **16**(1):153. DOI: 10.1186/s12916-018-1128-1

[8] Cheng HR, Walker LO, Tseng YF, Lin PC. Post-partum weight retention in women in Asia. A systematic review. Obesity Reviews. 2011;**12**(10):770-780

[9] Institute of Medicine. Dietary Reference Intakes for Energy, Carbohydrate, Fiber, Fat, Fatty Acids, Cholesterol, Protein, and Amino Acids. Washington, DC: The National Academies Press; 2005

[10] Kominiarek MA, Rajan P. Nutrition recommendations in pregnancy and lactation. The Medical Clinics of North America. 2016;**100**(6):1199-1215

[11] Brown LS. Nutrition requirements during pregnancy. In: Sharlin J, Edelstein J, editors. Essentials of Life Cycle Nutrition. USA: Jones & Bartlett Learning Publish; 2011. pp. 1-24. ISBN: 9780763777920

[12] Oteng-Ntim E, Varma R, Croker H, Poston L, Doyle P. Lifestyle interventions for overweight and obese pregnant women to improve pregnancy outcome: Systematic review and meta-analysis. BMC Medicine. 2012;**10**:47

[13] Goodnight W, Newman R. Society of Maternal-Fetal Medicine. Optimal nutrition for improved twin pregnancy outcome. Obstetrics and Gynecology. 2009;**114**(5):1121-1134

[14] Institute of Medicine. Dietary Reference Intakes: The Essential Guide to Nutrient Requirements. Washington DC: The National Academies Press; 2006

[15] Lacroix M et al. Lower adiponectin levels at first trimester of pregnancy are associated with increased insulin

resistance and higher risk of developing gestational diabetes mellitus. Diabetes Care. 2013;**36**(6):1577-1583

[16] Nguyen CL, Pham NM, Binns CW, Duong DV, Lee AL. Prevalence of gestational diabetes mellitus in eastern and southeastern Asia. A systematic review and meta-analysis. Journal Diabetes Research. 2018;**2018**:6536974. DOI: 10.1155/2018/6536974

[17] Dias S, Pheiffer C, Abrahams Y, Rheeder P, Adam S. Molecular biomarkers for gestational diabetes mellitus. International Journal of Molecular Sciences. 2018;**19**(10):2926

[18] Kang YE, Kim JM, Joung KH, et al. The roles of adipokines, proinflammatory cytokines, and adipose tissue macrophages in obesity-associated insulin resistance in modest obesity and early metabolic dysfunction. PLoS One. 2016;**11**(4):e0154003

[19] Makki K, Froguel P, Wolowczuk I. Adipose tissue in obesity-related inflammation and insulin resistance: Cells, cytokines, and chemokines. ISRN Inflammation. 2013;**2013**:139239

[20] Romeo GR, Lee J, Shoelson SE. Metabolic syndrome, insulin resistance, and roles of inflammation-mechanisms and therapeutic targets. Arteriosclerosis, Thrombosis, and Vascular Biology. 2012;**32**(8):1771-1776

[21] Tamori Y, Sakaue H, Kasuga M. RBP4, an unexpected adipokine. Nature Medicine. 2006;**12**:30-31

[22] Sudharshana Murthy KA, Bhandiwada A, Chandan SL, Gowda SL, Sindhusree G. Evaluation of oxidative stress and proinflammatory cytokines in gestational diabetes mellitus and their correlation with pregnancy outcome. Indian Journal of Endocrinology and Metabolism. 2018; **22**(1):79-84

[23] Liong S, Lappas M. Endoplasmic reticulum stress is increased in adipose tissue of women with gestational diabetes. PLoS One. 2015;**10**(4): e0122633

[24] American Diabetes Association. Standards of Medical Care in Diabetes. Diabetes Care. 2018;**41**(Supplement 1): S13-S27

[25] Eades CE, Cameron DM, Evans JMM. Prevalence of gestational diabetes mellitus in Europe. A meta-analysis. Diabetes Research and Clinical Practice. 2017;**129**:173-181. DOI: 10.1016/j.diabres.2017.03.030

[26] Sweeting AN, Ross GP, Hyett J, et al. Gestational diabetes mellitus in early pregnancy: Evidence for poor pregnancy outcomes despite treatment. Diabetes Care. 2016;**39**(1):75-81. DOI: 10.2337/dc15-0433

[27] Kim C, Ferrara A, editors. Gestational Diabetes During and After Pregnancy. New York: Springer; 2010

[28] American Diabetes Association. Classification and diagnosis of diabetes. Diabetes Care. 2017;**40** (Suppl.1):S11-S24

[29] The American College of Obstetricians and Gynecologists (ACOG). Gestational Diabetes Mellitus. ACOG Practice Bulletin No. 180. USA: The American College of Obstetricians and Gynecologists; 2017

[30] Farrar D. Hyperglycemia in pregnancy: Prevalence, impact, and management challenges. International Journal of Women's Health. 2016;**8**: 519-527. DOI: 10.2147/IJWH.S102117

[31] Shepherd E, Gomersall JC, Tieu J, Han S, Crowther CA, Middleton P. Combined diet and exercise interventions for preventing gestational diabetes mellitus. The Cochrane

Database of Systematic Reviews. 2017; **11**:CD010443. DOI: 10.1002/14651858. CD010443.pub

[32] Han S, Middleton P, Shepherd E, Van Ryswyk E, Crowther CA. Different types of dietary advice for women with gestational diabetes mellitus. The Cochrane Database of Systematic Reviews. 2017;**2**:CD009275. DOI: 10.1002/14651858.CD009275.pub3

[33] Khooshehchin TE, Keshavarz Z, Afrakhteh M, Shakibazadeh E, Faghihzadeh S. Perceived needs in women with gestational diabetes: A qualitative study. Electronic Physician Journal. 2016;**8**(12):3412-3420. DOI: 10.19082/3412

[34] Letherby G, Stephen N, Stenhouse E. Pregnant women with pre-existing diabetes: Family support in managing the pregnancy process. Human Fertility. 2012;**15**(4):200-204

[35] Magon N, Seshiah V. Gestational diabetes mellitus: Non-insulin management. Indian Journal of Endocrinology and Metabolism. 2011; **15**(4):284-293

[36] Reader DM. Medical nutrition therapy and lifestyle interventions. Diabetes Care. 2007;**20**(3):S188-S193

[37] American Diabetes Association. Nutrition principles and recommendations in diabetes. Diabetes Care. 2004;**27**(Supp. 1):S36-S46

[38] Agarwal MM, Dhatt GS, Shah SM. Gestational diabetes mellitus: Simplifying the international association of diabetes and pregnancy diagnostic algorithm using fasting plasma glucose. Diabetes Care. 2010;**33**(9):2018-2020

[39] Wylie-Rosett J, Aebersold K, Conlon B, Isasi CR, Ostrovsky NW. Health effects of low-carbohydrate diets: Where should new research go? Current Diabetes Reports. 2013;**13**(2):271-278

[40] Hernandez TL, Van Pelt RE, Anderson MA, et al. A higher-complex carbohydrate diet in gestational diabetes mellitus achieves glucose targets and lowers postprandial lipids: A randomized crossover study. Diabetes Care. 2014;**37**(5):1254-1262

[41] Thomas AM, Gutierrez YM. Gestational Diabetes Mellitus. Chicago, IL: American Dietetic Association; 2005

[42] Dornhorst A, Frost G. The principles of dietary management of gestational diabetes: Reflection on current evidence. Journal of Human Nutrition and Dietetics. 2002;**15**: 145-156. Quiz 157-149

[43] Shin D, Lee KW, Song WO. Dietary patterns during pregnancy are associated with risk of gestational diabetes mellitus. Nutrients. 2015;**7**(11): 9369-9382

[44] Fitzgerald MA, McCouch SR, Hall RD. Not just a grain of rice: The quest for quality. Trends in Plant Science. 2009;**14**:133-139

[45] Ranawana DV, Henry CJK, Lightowler HJ, Wang D. Glycaemic index of some commercially available rice and rice products in Great Britain. International Journal of Food Sciences and Nutrition. 2009;**60**:99-110

[46] Yusof BNM, Talib RA, Karim NA. Glycaemic index of eight types of commercial rice in Malaysia. Malaysian Journal of Nutrition. 2005;**11**(2):151-163

[47] Ishak WRW, Muda WAMW, Bakar NA, Malik VS, Willett WC, Frank BH, et al. Glycaemic index of commercially available brown rice in East Coast of Peninsular Malaysia. Middle-East Journal of Scientific Research. 2016; **24**(4):1430-1435

[48] Eleazu CO. The concept of low glycemic index and glycemic load foods as panacea for typ. 2 diabetes mellitus;

prospects, challenges and solutions. African Health Sciences. 2016;**16**(2): 468-479

[49] Arner P, Andersson DP, Bäckdahl J, Dahlman I, Rydén M. Weight gain and impaired glucose metabolism in women are predicted by inefficient subcutaneous fat cell lipolysis. Cell Metabolism. 2018;**28**(1):45-54.e3

[50] Bray GA, Lovejoy JC, Smith SR. The influence of different fats and fatty acids on obesity, insulin resistance and inflammation. Journal of Nutrition. 2002;**132**:2488-2491

[51] Riccardia G, Giaccob R, Rivellesea AA. Dietary fat, insulin sensitivity and the metabolic syndrome. Clinical Nutrition. 2004;**23**(4):447-456

[52] Moon HS, Dalamaga M, Kim SY, et al. Leptin's role in lipodystrophic and nonlipodystrophic insulin-resistant and diabetic individuals. Endocrine Reviews. 2013;**34**(3):377-412

[53] Zhou YJ, Tang YS, Song YL, Li A, Zhou H, Li Y. Saturated fatty acid induces insulin resistance partially through nucleotide-binding oligomerization domain 1 signaling pathway in adipocytes. Chinese Medical Sciences Journal. 2013;**28**(4):211-217

[54] Hernandez TL, Anderson MA, Chartier-Logan C, Friedman JE, Barbour LA. Strategies in the nutritional management of gestational diabetes. Clinical Obstetrics and Gynecology. 2013;**56**(4):803-815

[55] Jamilian M, Samimi M, Mirhosseini N, et al. A randomized double-blinded, placebo-controlled trial investigating the effect of fish oil supplementation on gene expression related to insulin action, blood lipids, and inflammation in gestational diabetes mellitus-fish oil supplementation and gestational diabetes. Nutrients. 2018;**10**(2):163. DOI: 10.3390/nu10020163

[56] Bodnar LM, Simhan HN, Catov JM, et al. Maternal vitamin D status and the risk of mild and severe preeclampsia. Epidemiology. 2014;**25**(2):207-214

[57] Niyazoglu M, Hatipoglu E, Aydogan B, Dellal F, Yavuz A, Hacioglu Y, et al. Relation of maternal vitamin D status with gestational diabetes mellitus and perinatal outcome. African Health Sciences. 2015;**15**:523-531

[58] Kim BH, Glanz K, Nehl EJ. Vitamin D beliefs and associations with sunburns, sun exposure, and sun protection. International Journal of Environmental Research and Public Health. 2012;**9**(7):2386-2395

[59] De-Regil LM, Palacios C, Lombardo LK, Pena-Rosas JP. Vitamin D supplementation for women during pregnancy (Review). Cochrane Database of Systematic Reviews. 2016;**1**: 1-124

[60] The Royal College of Obstetricians and Gynaecologists. Vitamin D in Pregnancy. Scientific Impact Paper No. 43. London: The Royal College of Obstetricians and Gynaecologists; 2014. https://www.rcog.org.uk/globalassets/documents/guidelines/scientific-impact-papers/vitamin_d_sip43_june14.pdf

[61] Goodnight W, Newman R. Optimal nutrition for improved twin pregnancy outcome. Obstetrics and Gynecology. 2009;**114**:1121-1134

[62] De-Regil LM, Palacios C, Ansary A, Kulier R, Peña-Rosas JP. Vitamin D supplementation for women during pregnancy. The Cochrane Database of Systematic Reviews. 2012;**2**(2): CD008873. DOI: 10.1002/14651858.CD008873.pub2

[63] Palacios C, Gonzalez L. Is vitamin D deficiency a major global public health problem? The Journal of Steroid

Biochemistry and Molecular Biology. 2014;**144**(Pt A):138-145

[64] Dovnik A, Mujezinovic F. The association of vitamin D levels with common pregnancy complications. Nutrients. 2018;**10**:867

[65] Tamura T, Picciano M. Folate and human reproduction. The American Journal of Clinical Nutrition. 2006;**83**: 993-1016

[66] Deave T, Johnson D, Ingram J. Transition to parenthood: The needs of parents in pregnancy and early parenthood. BMC Pregnancy and Childbirth. 2008;**8**:30. DOI: 10.1186/ 1471-2393-8-30

[67] Centre for Maternal and Child Enquires and Royal College of Obstetricians and Gynaecologists Joint Guideline: Management of women with obesity in pregnancy. London: Centre for Maternal and Child Enquiries; 2010

[68] Weiser MJ, Butt CM, Mohajeri MH. Docosahexaenoic acid and cognition throughout the lifespan. Nutrients. 2016;**8**(2):99

[69] Emmett R, Akkersdyk S, Yeatman H, Meyer BJ. Expanding awareness of docosahexaenoic acid during pregnancy. Nutrients. 2013;**5**:1098-1109

[70] U.S. EPA. Exposure Factors Handbook 2011 Edition (Final Report). Washington, DC: U.S. Environmental Protection Agency; 2011. EPA/600/R-09/052F

[71] European Commission. Information Note, Subject: Methyl Mercury in Fish and Fishery Products. https://www.efsa.europa.eu/sites/default/files/assets/af040608-ax9.pdf [Accessed October, 12, 2018]

[72] The United States Environmental Protection Agency (EPA). EPA-FDA Fish Advice: Technical Information. https://www.epa.gov/fish-tech/epa-fda-fish-advice-technical-information [Accessed October 12, 2018]

[73] Knowles TG, Farrington D, Kestin SC. Mercury in UK imported fish and shellfish and UK-farmed fish and their products. Food Additives & Contaminants. 2003;**20**(9):813-818

[74] Farah N, Kennedy C, Turner C, O'Dwyer V, Kennelly MM, Turner MJ. Maternal obesity and pre-pregnancy folic acid supplementation. Obesity Facts. 2013;**6**:211-215. DOI: 10.1159/ 000350393

[75] Zhang Z, Fulgoni VL, Kris-Etherton PM, Mitmesser SH. Dietary Intakes of EPA and DHA Omega-3 Fatty Acids among US Childbearing-Age and Pregnant Women: An Analysis of NHANES 2001-2014. Nutrients. 2018; **10**(4):416. DOI:10.3390/nu10040416

Chapter 5

Hydrops Fetalis

Renuka Sekar

Abstract

The abnormal accumulation of fluid in two or more fetal space and in some cases is associated with placental edema and polyhydramnios. This can be seen in all trimesters. It is classified as immune and nonimmune fetal hydrops. Immune hydrops fetalis-rhesus alloimmunization and other blood group antibodies cause hemolytic disease of the newborn. Nonimmune hydrops fetalis can be largely divided as fetal, maternal, placental and idiopathic. Pathophysiology, investigations, treatment and counseling are outlined.

Keywords: fetal hydrops, hydrops fetalis, immune hydrops, nonimmune fetal hydrops, pathophysiology

1. Introduction

Hydrops fetalis or fetal hydrops is an abnormal fluid collection in two or more fetal compartments. This includes skin edema (>5 mm), ascites, pleural, and pericardial effusion. In some, this may be associated with the placental edema (placental thickness > 4 cm in the second trimester and >6 mm in the third trimester) [1] and polyhydramnios [2].

Hydrops fetalis is a serious fetal condition usually identified by ultrasound examination. Very rarely, subtle collection of fluid may be missed on ultrasound scan. Historically, hydrops fetalis was due to rhesus alloimmunisation, especially prior to prophylactic anti-D administration in the developed countries, although this may not be the case in many developing countries.

1.1 Terminologies

Hydrops fetalis is the abnormal accumulation of fluid within the fetal skin, abdomen, pleural space, and or pericardium [1, 3].

Edema/anasarca is the term for fluid accumulation in the subcutaneous tissues of the skin.

Excess fluid accumulation within the peritoneal cavity is frequently referred to as ascites.

1.2 Epidemiology

The precise incidence of hydrops fetalis is difficult as some cases spontaneously resolve or diagnosis is not seen until fetal demise or miscarriage. The overall incidence of fetal hydrops reported in the literature is between 1 in 1500 and 1 in 3000 pregnancies [4].

With the advent of anti-D immunoglobulin, the incidence and mortality due to immune hydrops fetalis have reduced with an increase in nonimmune fetal hydrops in about 90% of cases [5–8].

The diagnosis of hydrops fetalis is usually made antenatally and is a challenging condition to counsel and is usually a preterminal manifestation of many different pathophysiological conditions.

A recent publication from a single centre in Australia showed that the overall survival from diagnosis was 27%. The perinatal mortality risk is high when infants are born with hydrops fetalis and is dependent on the underlying diagnosis.

2. Classification

Hydrops fetalis is broadly classified into immune and nonimmune.

2.1 Immune fetal hydrops

Immune hydrops fetalis is due to red cell antibodies. There are many red cell antibodies of which rhesus D, c, and E are the commonest. The incidence of Rh D antibodies is reducing secondary due to the widespread use of anti-D at least in the developed countries. There appears to be an increase in other red cell antibodies that are now commonly associated with immune hydrops fetalis that can cause hemolytic disease of the newborn. These are kell antibodies, Duffy, and other red cell antibodies. Lewis and p antibodies rarely cause hemolytic disease of the newborn. The mechanism of fetal hydrops is secondary to fetal anemia. Fetal anemia is due to direct red cell destruction by the red cell antibodies that cross the placenta, especially if the baby has a different blood group and type to the mother. Anemia causes high output cardiac failure and fetal hydrops.

In the Caucasian population, about 85% are rhesus (Rh) positive, which leaves about 15% Rh negative. When the mother is Rh negative and has never been sensitized before (no previous pregnancy, miscarriage, termination of pregnancy, or ectopic pregnancy), the sensitization event happens with the first pregnancy if the partner is positive. A sensitization event can happen spontaneously during pregnancy (feto maternal hemorrhage) and in labour or during an event such as maternal trauma, abruption, invasive procedures, antepartum hemorrhage, and external cephalic version. During these events, anti-D must be administered in Rh-negative women with an Rh positive partner. When possible, partner testing for both phenotype and genotype of his blood group must be requested. Currently, the widespread use of free fetal DNA in the detection of fetal D gene is helpful in identifying the Rh status of the fetus from maternal blood sample performed after 10 weeks of gestation. Amniocentesis can be performed to assess the fetal Rh D status as well; this will again increase the sensitization during pregnancy.

Hydrops fetalis that develop in the absence of red cell hemolysis is termed as nonimmune fetal hydrops (NIFH) and was first described by Dr. Potter in 1943. The reported incidence of nonimmune fetal hydrops (NIFH) is 1 in 2000–3000 pregnancies [4, 5]. These result in about 3% of perinatal mortality and 50% diagnosed in utero will result in fetal demise and 50% of live born will not survive the neonatal period.

2.2 Nonimmune fetal hydrops (NIFH)

There are many causes for nonimmune fetal hydrops. In the past, many were thought to be idiopathic. Recent literature review shows that a cause can be identified prenatally in 65% of cases and up to 85% postnatally [9]. They are broadly divided as maternal, fetal, placental, and idiopathic causes.

2.2.1 Maternal

Hemoglobinopathies (both alpha and beta thalassemia) are caused especially when both parents are carriers. Alpha thalassemia can cause severe fetal hydrops early in pregnancy, especially Barts [10] hemoglobinopathy (4 gene deletion)—hemolysis is the cause of fetal hydrops, fetomaternal hemorrhage (abruption), and maternal hemolytic anemia.

Infection—some maternal infections can cause fetal infection and affect neural development, e.g., cytomegalovirus, toxoplasmosis, parvovirus [11] (erythrogenic), syphilis, and Zika virus.

Maternal antibodies—anti-Ro and La antibodies can be positive in mothers with autoimmune disorders such as systemic lupus erythematosis, rheumatoid arthritis. These mothers are tested for other antibodies including antiphospholipid and extractable nuclear antibodies (Ro and La). These antibodies cross the placenta and in 6% of cases can cause congenital heart block in the fetus as they affect the purkinje fibers of the heart. With a very low heart rate, the fetus is at increased risk of developing hydrops [12, 13] (low cardiac output and heart failure).

Neonatal alloimmune thrombocytopenia and idiopathic thrombocytopenia—in neonatal alloimmune thrombocytopenia (NAIT), due to incompatible platelet antibodies (human platelet antibody A1A and 5A) between maternal and paternal platelets, there is production of antibodies against maternal platelets. The risk of neonatal thrombocytopenia is very high, 85–100%. These IgG antibodies cross the placenta and destroy fetal platelets causing anemia and fetal hydrops. Unlike rhesus alloimmunisation where the first pregnancy is less likely to be affected when there was no preceding sensitizing event, NAIT affects the first pregnancy (diagnosis is made after the affected pregnancy) and increases the risk for subsequent pregnancies.

When there is maternal idiopathic thrombocytopenia, the risk of fetal thrombocytopenia is low 1–2%, fetal monitoring is recommended both antenatally and intrapartum. The risk of fetal thrombocytopenia is high when maternal platelets fall below 20×10^6.

2.2.2 Placental

Placental chorioangiomas are tumors of the placenta and is usually a pathological diagnosis. When the size of the chorioangiomas is over 5 cms and the cord insertion is close to the chorioangioma, there is an increased vascular turbulence leading to microangiopathic anemia leading to fetal hydrops and polyhydramnios.

Monochorionic twin pregnancies—especially in 15% of monochorionic diamniotic twin gestations, there is unbalanced vascular communication between the twins leading to unbalanced transfusion where one of the twins can be hydropic (recipient) or polycythemic, while the other can be anemic. Untreated twin-to-twin transfusion [14] leads to fetal hydrops in the recipient and fetal demise in one twin, which can in turn result in the death of the other twin as well.

2.2.3 Fetal

There are many fetal conditions that can give rise to fetal hydrops, which can be broadly classified as:

1. chromosomal—trisomy and 45XO (Turner's syndrome) [15]

2. structural

- fetal tumors of the face (epignathus) and neck
- cardiac (cardiomyopathies, tumors-rhabdomyomas, myocarditis, and abnormal fetal heart rates such as both fetal tachy and bradyarrhythmias)
- thoracic—pulmonary airway malformations [16] (microcystic or macrocystic) especially with mediastinal shift, bronchopulmonary sequestration, congenital hyperinflation obstructive airway syndrome, and primary lymphatic anomaly
- congenital diaphragmatic hernias—especially with mediastinal shift
- abdomen—tumors or large cysts in fetal abdomen, bowel dilatation, or obstruction/volvulus, meconium peritonitis
- sacrococcygeal teratomas—these tumors cause anemia secondary to high-output cardiac failure
- dental hemangiomas, arteriovenous malformations (AVM's), absent ductus venosus, and umbilical cord varix
- skeletal dysplasias
- cystic hygromas and lymphatic obstruction

3. fetal infections

   - toxoplasma, rubella, cytomegalovirus, herpes virus, syphilis, and parvovirus are the common fetal infections. Parvovirus is highly erythrogenic, and the resulting fetal anemia is due to failed erythropoiesis. There is an estimated 1–2% risk of seroconversion in pregnancy that increases to 10% during epidemics. There is still a fetal loss rate of 3–10% depending on gestational age of exposure

4. hematological—secondary to congenital leukemia or red cell erythrogenic abnormalities (Blackfan-Diamond syndrome and congenital dyserythropoiesis)

5. fetal metabolic abnormalities, most of them are autosomal recessive—G6PD deficiencies

6. fetal genetic or neurologic syndromes

7. miscellaneous—severe fetal growth restriction, fetal akinesia, or hypomobility syndromes

8. idiopathic—30–50% of fetal hydrops

Fetal tachyarrhythmia includes supraventricular tachycardia, fetal atrial fibrillation, or flutter. In total, 90% of fetal tachyarrhythmia is due to fetal supraventricular tachyarrhythmia. Atrial flutter (FHR > 300 bpm) and fibrillation are less common. When fetal heart rates are above 220 bpm, there is reduced diastolic filling with reduced ejection fraction and cardiac output. This in turn results in poor perfusion, reduced oxygenation, and elevated CVP and hepatic congestion. The risk of fetal hydrops is inversely related to gestational age, and this could be related to immaturity of fetal myocardium [17].

Fetal bradyarrhythmias are due to congenital heart block, and fetal hydrops is secondary to low cardiac output and inadequate oxygen perfusion and also to venous congestion. The risk is higher when FHR is less than 95 bpm and often when <65 bpm.

Congenital structural anomalies of the heart may predispose to high output failure and may be associated with other chromosomal or structural anomalies [18].

Heritable hemoglobinopathies are usually autosomal recessive, and testing for this is done is either done pre or antenatally. Fetal anemia causes high output cardiac failure and increased central venous pressure, leading to fetal hydrops. Antiplatelet antibodies cross the placenta and destroy fetal platelets similar to rhesus alloimmunisation, resulting in fetal anemia and hydrops.

Fetal infection that crosses the placenta usually causes myocarditis, suppresses erythropoiesis, causes hemolysis, and hepatitis. Examples of fetal infection are toxoplasma, cytomegalovirus, rubella, herpes virus, syphilis, parvovirus and others include coxsackie virus, *Listeria monocytogenes*.

Hydrops fetalis is associated with more than 75 inborn errors of metabolism, genetic syndromes, and chromosomal abnormalities. The inheritance is usually autosomal recessive with some conditions that could be X linked.

Cystic hygromas are usually associated with aberration in lymphatic drainage. They are usually seen as cystic spaces in the fetal neck, but can also be seen in fetal thorax or abdomen. These findings can be associated with 45XO (Turner's syndrome) [6] and are usually seen in aborted fetuses. There are some cases of spontaneous resolution of cystic hygromas, but prognosis is usually poor (90–95% mortality) especially when associated with hydrops fetalis even with normal karyotype. The differential diagnoses include Noonan syndrome and multiple pterygium syndrome.

Thoracic and abdominal tumors, by way of their size and location, obstruct both venous and lymphatic return to the fetal heart, causing fetal hydrops.

In some tumors such as sacrococcygeal teratomas [19] or chorioangiomas, the resulting fetal hydrops is not only due to the size of the tumor but also due to the increased vascularity in them behaving like an arteriovenous malformation, leading to high output cardiac failure, and microangiopathic fetal anemia.

Isolated pleural effusion, unilateral or bilateral, is seen without progression to fetal hydrops, especially with abnormal lymphatic development [20].

3. Pathophysiology

There have been many hypotheses for fetal hydrops. Distribution of body water is between the intracellular (blood and tissues) and extracellular (plasma, interstitial space, and transcellular) space.

The basic mechanism is an abnormal fluid movement between plasma and tissues and the imbalance between the interstitial production and lymphatic return [21].

Four main theories have been postulated:

1. heart failure or obstruction to venous return causes increase in hydrostatic capillary pressure,

2. hepatic congestion causing reduced production of albumin causing reduced plasma oncotic pressure,

3. lymphatic flow obstruction,

4. damage to peripheral capillary integrity.

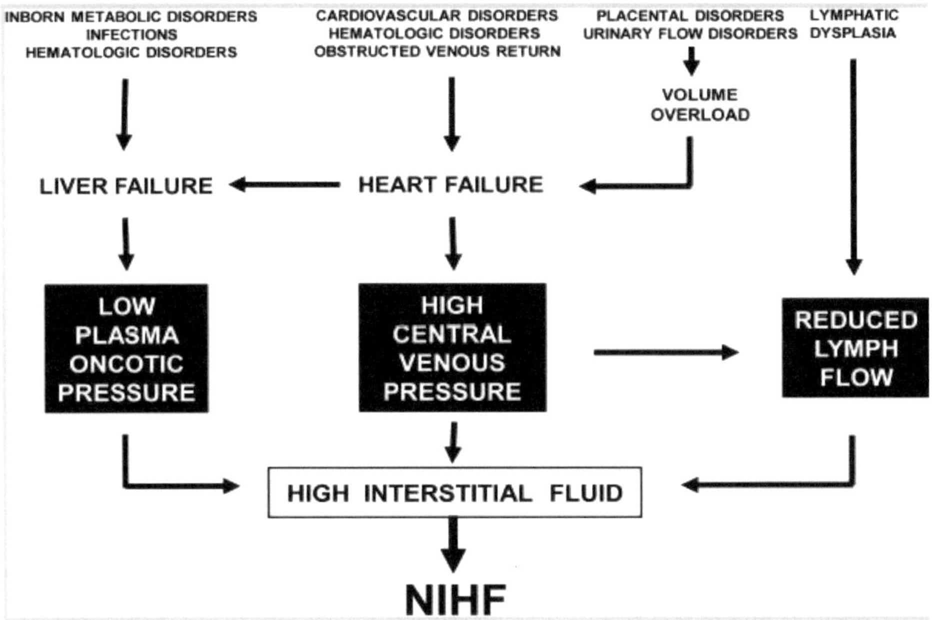

Figure 1.
Flow chart of possible pathophysiology in NIFH [6].

Fluid accumulation may be due to congestive cardiac failure, obstruction to the lymphatic flow, or reduced oncotic pressure. The fetus has greater capillary permeability and an interstitial compartment that can accommodate extra fluid.

When there is fetal hypoxia, there is redistribution to the vital organs such as brain, heart, and adrenals. There is reduced blood flow to fetal kidneys and gut. The reduced renal blood flow activates the renin angiotensin system (RAS) to enhance cardiac output. This also increases the venous pressure and thereby increases in interstitial fluid accumulation.

Due to reduced hepatic blood flow and increase in extramedullary hematopoiesis, there is reduction in albumin production causing hypoalbuminemia, thereby reducing the oncotic pressure and causing fluid shift. Many animal models have been studied in order to understand hydrops. The largest systematic review by Bellini et al. [6] also illustrated the possible pathophysiological causes of NIFH (**Figure 1**).

With fetal hydrops, there is a risk of maternal mirror syndrome (Ballantyne's syndrome) in some patients, where the mother develops edema similar to the hydropic fetus.

Mirror syndrome represents a form of preeclampsia characterized by edema (90%), high blood pressure (60%), and proteinuria (40%) of cases [22–25]. The incidence is unclear and may not be reported. Review of literature shows a maternal mortality of about 20% secondary to pulmonary edema. With treatment for fetal hydrops, maternal symptoms have noted to resolve.

The imbalance between the angiogenic and antiangiogenic factors that are implicated in severe preeclampsia is also thought to be the underlying pathogenesis of this condition. When the underlying NIFH cannot be treated and when there are ongoing symptoms of maternal mirror syndrome, delivery is indicated.

4. Investigations

Maternal blood tests—the first line of investigation would be to rule out immune hydrops fetalis.

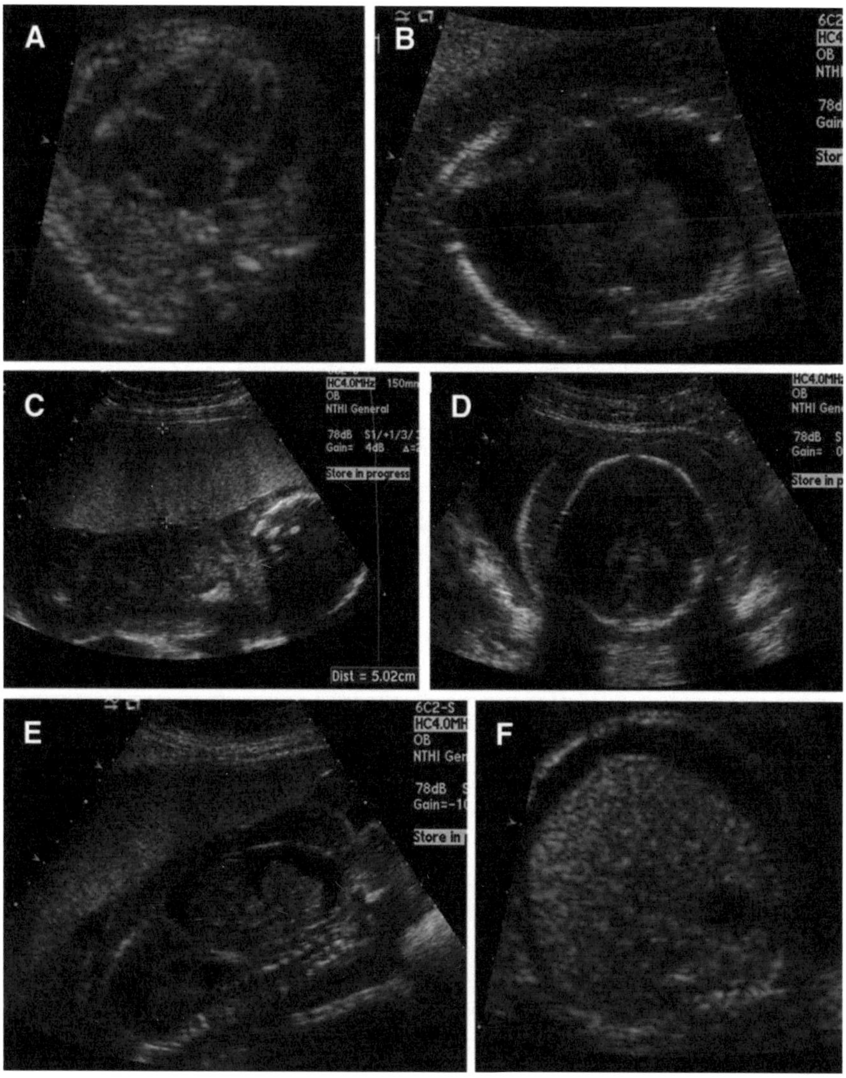

Figure 2.
Ultrasound findings fetal hydrops [1]. (A) Pericardial effusions, (B) pleural effusions; note: midline heart anterior to small lungs with bilateral effusions, (C) placental thickening, with placenta measuring >4 mm in thickness, (D) skin thickening at level of fetal skull, (E) ascites, sagittal, with free-floating loops of bowel surrounded by ascites, and (F) ascites in upper abdomen, at level of fetal liver and stomach [1].

Maternal rhesus status, antibodies, full blood count, Kleihauer-Betke test, and indirect Coombs test are requested.

The other blood tests are for nonimmune hydrops fetalis.

Hemoglobin electrophoresis is requested to rule out thalassemia, both alpha and beta. This screen is especially important in Mediterranean, Indian, and Asian ethnic groups.

TORCHS+P serology (toxoplasma, rubella, cytomegalovirus, herpes, syphilis, and parvovirus).

If fetal heart rate is lower than 100 bpm, anti-Ro and La antibodies to be requested.

Maternal serum electrolytes and liver function tests, including urinary PCR, are recommended to rule out maternal mirror syndrome. When fetal hydrops is associated with abnormal placenta, triploidy or partial molar pregnancy cannot be ruled out; hence, serum beta-HCG and thyroid function tests are performed in this situation.

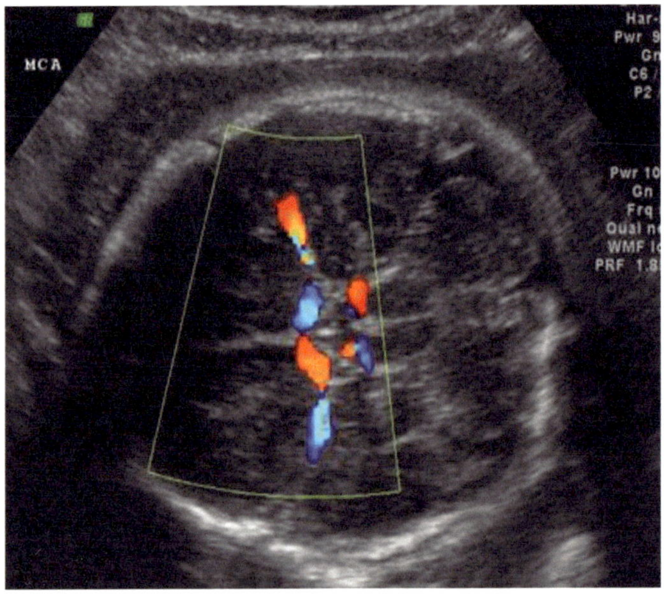

Figure 3.
Transverse section of fetal head showing middle cerebral artery—Google images.

A detailed tertiary ultrasound of the fetus/fetuses is recommended including amniotic fluid volume and Doppler studies looking for fetal anemia.

Fetal tertiary ultrasound is the key to diagnose most of the above-mentioned fetal structural abnormalities. A thorough assessment including fetal weight, morphology, amniotic fluid volume, and placental morphology are recommended.

Fetal heart rate documentation is vital to rule out both tachy and brady arrhythmias.

Fetal dopplers including umbilical artery, vein, ductus venosus, tricuspid regurgitation, and middle cerebral artery peak systolic velocity (MCA PSV) measurements are very helpful in the investigation of hydrops fetalis.

The middle cerebral artery Doppler known as MCA peak systolic velocity is a good noninvasive measure of fetal anemia. With fetal anemia and possible hypoxia, velocity of blood flow to the fetal brain increases. When the MCA PSV is above 1.5 multiples of the median (MoM), there is a high risk of fetal anemia. The false-positive rate of this measurement is around 10% and increases after 35 weeks of gestation (**Figures 2** and **3**).

Invasive testing such as amniocentesis and amniodrainage [26] is discussed and performed under ultrasound guidance. Maternal rhesus status is checked so that the patient is given anti-D when not sensitized.

The amniotic fluid is sent for chromosome tests—fluorescent in situ hybridization (FISH), chromosomal microarray, rasopathy, or hydrops panel including Noonan's syndrome, lysosomal storage disease and in some centres whole exome sequencing. Polymerase chain reaction (PCR) from the amniotic fluid is sent for fetal infection such as TORCHS+parvovirus' DNA for specific conditions if known.

When there is evidence of fetal pleural effusion, either a pleural tap or insertion of a pleuroamniotic shunt is inserted to drain the pleural effusion/effusions [27]. The sample is also sent for lymphocytes apart from infection and karyotype.

The presence of fetal sacrococcygeal teratoma is confirmed, and fetal magnetic resonance imaging (MRI) may be required to identify the intrapelvic extension.

5. Management of NIFH

Transfer to maternal and fetal medicine unit is recommended. The outcome for most cases of NIFH is poor unless there is a treatable cause. Women are not only extensively counseled [28] regarding outcomes with NIFH, but also for risks such as polyhydramnios (29%) and preterm labour (66%). When there is an ongoing maternal symptom with severe polyhydramnios, amniodrainage is recommended.

The outcome usually falls into

1. Treatable cause of NIFH—fetal tachyarrhythmia's (antiarrhythmic medications), fetal anemia secondary to parvovirus B19 infection (in utero fetal transfusion), large macrocystic congenital pulmonary airway malformation (CPAM) (shunt or antenatal corticosteroids), twin-twin transfusion syndrome (TTTS) (laser photocoagulation), and twin-reversed arterial perfusion (TRAP) (selective radiofrequency ablation), fetal sacrococcygeal teratoma's with an identified fetal vessel may benefit from radiofrequency or laser ablation.

2. Lethal prognosis—termination of pregnancy or palliative care should be offered.

3. Idiopathic—with uncertain to poor prognosis.

When NIFH is identified before viability with no identifiable cause, pregnancy termination should be discussed and offered. Termination of pregnancy should be considered when associated with maternal complications such as maternal mirror syndrome. Antepartum surveillance is usually recommended depending on gestational age at diagnosis and the underlying cause of NIFH. Once the underlying cause of fetal hydrops is treated, ongoing surveillance is important to plan delivery. Mode of delivery depends on underlying etiology, gestational age, and maternal well-being. Vaginal delivery is considered when there is a lethal condition with no fetal monitoring. Cesarean delivery is recommended in all other conditions. When there is moderate to severe pleural effusion, drainage prior to delivery may help in the neonatal period. Elective preterm delivery is not recommended unless indicated, as this does not improve neonatal outcomes.

In a recent review of a 12-year retrospective cohort from a single centre [9], the overall survival from diagnosis was 27% increasing to 55% if born alive.

The long-term prognosis of survivors of NIFH also depends on underlying etiology. Following parvovirus B19 infection with fetal anemia and transfusion, there appears to be some neurological sequelae in about 30% of babies [29]. This could be a direct consequence of parvovirus infection with fetal anemia or transfusion.

Fetuses with supraventricular tachycardia, some babies may develop Wolf Parkinson White syndrome later in life [30].

6. Conclusion

Ultrasound is the diagnostic tool for antenatal diagnosis of hydrops fetalis including all fetal Doppler studies. A detailed history and examination of the mother is very important. Serological testing for perinatal fetal infections and maternal antibodies helps in the workup of fetal hydrops. Tertiary referral to a maternal and fetal medicine unit is highly recommended. Outcome for babies with no antenatal diagnosis is very guarded to poor with increased neonatal morbidity and mortality.

Author details

Renuka Sekar
Royal Brisbane and Women's Hospital Brisbane, Queensland, Australia

*Address all correspondence to: renuka.sekar@health.qld.gov.au

References

[1] Norton ME, Chauhan SP, Dashe JS, Society for Maternal-Fetal Medicine (SMFM). Society for maternal-fetal medicine (SMFM) clinical guideline #7: Nonimmune hydrops fetalis. American Journal of Obstetrics and Gynecology. 2015;**212**:127-139

[2] Skoll MA, Sharland GK, Allan LD. Is the ultrasound definition of fluid collections in non-immune hydrops fetalis helpful in defining the underlying cause or predicting outcome? Ultrasound in Obstetrics & Gynecology. 1991;**1**:309-312

[3] Désilets V, Audibert F, Society of Obstetrician and Gynaecologists of Canada. Investigation and management of non-immune fetal hydrops. Journal of Obstetrics and Gynaecology Canada. 2013;**35**:923-936

[4] Hutchison AA, Drew JH, Yu VY, et al. Nonimmunologic hydrops fetalis: A review of 61 cases. Obstetrics and Gynecology. 1982;**59**:347-352

[5] Graves GR, Baskett TF. Nonimmune hydrops fetalis: Antenatal diagnosis and management. American Journal of Obstetrics and Gynecology. 1984;**148**:563-565

[6] Bellini C, Hennekam RC, Fulcheri E, et al. Etiology of nonimmune hydrops fetalis: A systematic review. American Journal of Medical Genetics Part A. 2009;**149A**:844-851

[7] Steurer MA, Peyvandi S, Baer RJ, et al. Epidemiology of live born infants with nonimmune hydrops fetalis-insights from a population-based dataset. The Journal of Pediatrics. 2017;**1**(87):182-188

[8] Pasman SA, Oepkes D, et al. Hypoalbuminemia: A cause of fetal hydrops? American Journal of Obstetrics and Gynecology. 2006;**194**(4):972-975

[9] Gilby DM et al. Outcomes following antenatal identification of hydrops fetalis: A single-center experience from 2001 to 2002. Archives of Disease in Childhood Fetal and Neonatal Edition. 2018;**0**:F1-F6

[10] Jomoui W, Sanchaisuriya K, et al. Genetic origin of α0-thalassemia (SEA deletion) in Southeast Asian populations and application to accurate prenatal diagnosis of Hb Bart's hydrops fetalis syndrome. Journal of Human Genetics. 2017;**62**(8):747-754

[11] Onroy A et al. Parvovirus B10 infection during pregnancy and risks to the fetus. Birth Defects Research. 2017;**109**(5):311-323

[12] Friedman DM et al. Prospective evaluation of fetuses with autoimmune associated congenital heart block followed in the PR interval and dexamethasone evaluation study (PRIDE) study. The American Journal of Cardiology. 2009;**103**:1102-1106

[13] Ciardulli A et al. Maternal steroid therapy for fetuses with immune-mediated complete atrioventricular block: A systematic review and meta-analysis. The Journal of Maternal-Fetal & Neonatal Medicine. 2017:1419182

[14] Van Den Wijingaard JP et al. Twin to twin transfusion syndrome modeling. Annals of the New York Academy of Sciences. 2017;**1101**:215-234

[15] Alpman A et al. Prenatlly diagnosed turner syndrome and cystic hygroma: Incidence and reasons for referrals. Fetal Diagnosis and Therapy. 2009;**25**:58-61

[16] Lee FL et al. Treatment of congenital pulmonary airway malformation induced hydrops fetalis via percutaneous scelrotherapy. Fetal Diagnosis and Therapy. 2012;**31**(4):264-268

[17] Moodley S et al. Postnatal outcome in patients with fetal tachycardia. Pediatric Cardiology. 2013;**34**:81-87

[18] Yuan SM. Cardiac etiologies of hydrops fetalis. Zeitschrift für Geburtshilfe und Neonatologie. 2017;**221**(2):67-72

[19] Van Mieghem T. Minimally invasive therapy for fetal sacrococcygeal teratoma: Case series and systematic review of the literature. Ultrasound in Obstetrics & Gynecology. 2014;**43**(6):611-619

[20] Williams IA et al. Is hydrops fetalis a manifestation of pulmonary edema caused by impaired lymphatic drainage? Ultrasound in Obstetrics & Gynecology. 2018;**31**(1):96-99

[21] Bellini C, Hennekam RC. Non-immune hydrops fetalis: A short review of etiology and pathophysiology. American Journal of Medical Genetics Part A. 2012;**158A**:597

[22] Braun T et al. Mirror syndrome: A systematic review of fetal associated conditions, maternal presentation and perinatal outcome. Fetal Diagnosis and Therapy. 2010;**27**:191-203

[23] Gedikbasi A et al. Preeclampsia due to fetal non-immune hydrops: Mirror syndrome and review of literature. Hypertension in Pregnancy. 2011;**30**:322-330

[24] Goa S et al. Normalization of angiognic imbalance after intra-uterine transfusion for mirror syndrome caused by parvovirus B19. Fetal Diagnosis and Therapy. 2013;**34**:176-179

[25] Llurba E et al. Angiogenic and antiangiogenic factors before and after resolution of maternal mirror syndrome. Ultrasound in Obstetrics & Gynecology. 2012;**40**:367-369

[26] Sandlin AT et al. Clinical relevance of sonographically estimated amniotic fluid volume: Polyhydramnios. Journal of Ultrasound in Medicine. 2013;**32**:851-863

[27] Nakayama A et al. The prognostic factors of hydrops fetalis with pleural effusion. Pediatrics International. 2017;**59**(10):1053-1057

[28] Santo S, Thilaganathan B, et al. Prenatal diagnosis of non-immune hydrops fetalis: What do we tell the parents? Prenatal Diagnosis. 2011;**31**(2):186-195

[29] Nassr AA et al. Outcome and treatment of antenatally diagnosed nonimmune hydrops fetalis. Fetal Diagnosis and Therapy. 2018;**43**(2):123-128

[30] Hahurij ND et al. Perinatal management and long-term cardiac outcome in fetal arrhythmia. Early Human Development. 2011;**87**:83-87

Section 3

Maternal Mortality

Chapter 6

Maternal and Fetal Complications Due to Decreased Nitric Oxide Synthesis during Gestation

Sonia Jurado, Kaelly Saraiva, Cauane Marceliano, Vanessa Souza and Izabela Vieira

Abstract

Nitric oxide (NO) is synthesized from L-arginine by the constitutive NO synthase in vascular endothelial cells and plays an important role in the regulation of blood pressure and coronary vasomotion. Normal pregnancy is associated with major adaptations in maternal cardiovascular function, which help the woman to accommodate the growing fetus. The vascular endothelium is stimulated during pregnancy to release increased amounts of NO, and the abnormality in the L-arginine NO pathway may play a role in the etiology of preeclampsia. The objective of this study is to discuss the importance of nitric oxide during gestation and the maternal and fetal complications associated with decreased NO synthesis during this period. Maternal arterial hypertension due to inhibition of nitric oxide synthesis during pregnancy impairs fetal development, mainly the reduction of the wall/lumen ratio of the cardiac and renal microvasculature as well as the reduction in the number of nephrons. These changes may contribute to the development of hypertension. Despite these findings, more studies are needed to understand the programming of fetal development, and the intrauterine environmental factors. influence this process.

Keywords: nitric oxide, pregnancy, preeclampsia, growth fetal, intrauterine environment

1. Introduction

Normal pregnancy is associated with intensive changes in the maternal cardiovascular system that enables adequate oxygen delivery and nutritive ingredients to the fetus. Physiological vascular adaptation (increased blood volume, increased cardiac minute volume, and reduced vascular resistance) is followed by increased endogenous production of nitric oxide (NO) and improved response of smooth muscles on the reaction of NO [1].

Nitric oxide is synthesized from L-arginine by the constitutive NO synthase in vascular endothelial cells and plays an important role in the regulation of blood pressure and coronary vasomotion. Abnormalities in its production and/or bioavailability are related to diseases such as hypertension, atherosclerosis, and disorders associated with angiogenesis [2].

In normal pregnancy, there is an increase in blood volume and maternal cardiac output, although a decrease in systemic blood pressure occurs. In addition, the responsiveness to various vasoconstrictors is attenuated. This is due to the contribution of nitric oxide (NO) to the vasodilatory phenomena of pregnancy [3].

Nitric oxide is a potent vasodilator and plays an important role in mild relaxation muscles and helps in the vasodilation of maternal blood flow. NO is derived from the amino acid L-arginine, which is in the proteins of all life forms. It is classified as a semi-essential or conditionally essential amino acid [4]. In addition to nitric oxide, other chemical mediators have been implicated in this phenomenon, including estradiol and prostacyclin [5].

Scrum NO concentration of the healthy pregnant women was significantly higher during the second and the third trimester of pregnancy in relation to control nonpregnant subjects [1]. Thus, increased production of nitric oxide by the endothelium contributes to the hemodynamic changes associated with normal pregnancy; conversely, a reduction in NO signaling has been observed in preeclampsia and in several forms of chronic hypertension [6, 7].

Preeclampsia is considered to be one of the most significant health problems in pregnancy, complicating 6–10% of all gestation over 20 weeks, 14–20% of multiple gestations, and 25% of patients with chronic hypertension and/or chronic renal disease [8, 9]. It is characterized of the symptomatic triad: hypertension (systolic pressure ≥ 140 mmHg and/or diastolic pressure ≥ 90 mmHg), proteinuria, and edema [10, 11]. This disease is one of the leading causes of fetal growth disorders, fetal morbidity and mortality, premature labor, and mother's death [4, 10].

Preeclampsia is a specific condition of gestation that involves the failure of several organs. The increase in blood pressure causes deleterious effects on several systems, especially the vascular, hepatic, renal, and cerebral. The complications observed in these systems may explain the high incidence of fetal and maternal mortality and morbidity, which makes preeclampsia one of the leading causes of maternal death in the world [1, 12].

It is interesting to note that there are some risk factors that increase the probability of a pregnant woman presenting with preeclampsia, such as hypertension and preexisting diabetes mellitus, obesity, and ethnicity [12].

Endothelial cell dysfunction can cause hypertension with its increased production of vasoconstrictor agents such as plasma endothelin or reduced release of vasodilator agents such as prostacyclin and NO [13].

Nitric oxide has been proposed as the physiological agent involved in this mechanism as it regulates feto-placental vascular permeability and resistance and platelet aggregation in the placenta. Maturation and development of the placenta is affected significantly by an epigenetic molecule such as nitric oxide which has been postulated to affect fetal programming and survival [14, 15].

The specific cause of NO increase during normal pregnancy is unknown, but it is suggested that increased shear stress during pregnancy stimulates the activity of the endothelial nitric oxide synthase (eNOS). Specifically in the placenta, the activity of this enzyme is important in the sense that NO synthesized locally maintains low vascular resistance, in addition to attenuating the action of vasoconstrictors [16].

The role of nitric oxide in the pathogenesis of preeclampsia was studied by Rachel et al. [4] who concluded that the circulating levels of nitrite are decreased in women with preeclampsia. One study showed that supplementation with L-arginine in women with preeclampsia lowered blood pressure through increased synthesis or bioavailability of nitric oxide [17].

Some studies point to the importance of nitric oxide to the outcome of pregnancy. Nitric oxide levels are altered in the blood serum of women who have had an abortion or ectopic pregnancy. The levels in recurrent abortions are decreased, leading to an increase in myometrial contraction, whereas in ectopic pregnancy levels are higher, leading to decreased uterine tube motility and ectopic implantation [18, 19].

2. Nitric oxide and uteroplacental circulation

The endothelial cells in the uteroplacental circulation play an important physiological role in the maintenance of vasodilation of placental vessels, since these are not innervated. These endothelial cells produce prostacyclin and nitric oxide, causing vasodilation and also preventing platelet aggregation and platelet adhesion to endothelial cells [19].

Nitric oxide (NO) regulates implantation and trophoblastic invasion as well as embryonic development [20]. In addition, vascular tone in the placenta is controlled by several vasoactive mediators, with NO being the most important [21].

Nitric oxide participates at the onset of placental vasculogenesis. The onset of vasculogenesis requires the expression of vascular endothelial growth factor (VEGF), the mitogenic effects of which are mediated by nitric oxide. There is no well-established level of NO required for adequate placental angiogenesis. Elevated levels of NO may prevent angiogenesis, and its effect on cell survival and proliferation depends on its concentration [22].

NO has an important role in facilitating pregnancy-induced expansive remodeling in the uterine circulation, especially in the larger arteries [7].

The NO signaling has an important role in the expansive circumferential gestational remodeling of the uterine circulation. It provides an interesting link to the theory that preeclampsia results from elevated levels of sFlt-1, a soluble receptor for vascular endothelial growth factor and placenta growth factor, in preeclamptic women [23].

An excess of soluble receptor would reduce the availability of these ligands to the maternal vascular wall and fetal growth retardation. The sFlt-1, when infused in pregnant rats, promotes glomerular proteinuria and endotheliosis, characteristics of the preeclampsia picture [24].

Since both placenta growth factor and vascular endothelial growth factor stimulate endothelial NO release, a reduction in their signaling would create a vasoconstrictor imbalance and increase peripheral resistance and blood pressure. Thus, a reduction in NO signaling also impacts vessel remodeling in a way that would further increase uterine vascular resistance. This effect on structure, combined with loss of function (vasodilation), would further mitigate the increases in uterine [7].

In addition to the decrease in the synthesis of nitric oxide in the uteroplacental circulation in preeclampsia, the endothelium-dependent relaxation in response to acetylcholine is impaired in preeclamptic arteries. Additionally, the increased plasma fibronectin levels in preeclampsia may reflect fibronectin which has been shed by injured endothelial cells. Furthermore, soluble circulating endothelial cell adhesion molecules such as soluble intercellular adhesion molecule-1 (sICAM-1), soluble vascular adhesion molecule-1 (sVCAM-1), and sE-selectin are significantly increased in preeclampsia compared to normal pregnancies. This suggests that there is an altered and pathological endothelial phenotype in preeclampsia [25].

3. Animal models for the study of nitric oxide during pregnancy

Animal models using rats or mice are very useful for the study of the pathogenesis, diagnosis, and treatment of preeclampsia. N-Nitro-L-arginine methyl ester (L-NAME) is an inhibitor of NO synthase, and it has been shown to promote arterial hypertension in pregnant rats [26, 27].

The administration of L-NAME in adult rats, in addition to causing hypertension [28], promotes cardiac and aortic tissue damage [29], proteinuria, and glomerular endotheliosis [30].

Several animals have already been used as models of experimental hypertension, such as rhesus monkeys, dogs, and sheep. Most of the experimental studies use rats and mice. In these animals, four categories of preeclampsia are produced: (i) animals with surgically induced reduced uteroplacental blood flow, (ii) animals with preclinical symptoms induced by drugs, (iii) genetic animal models, and (iv) animals with preexisting hypertension developing preeclampsia [31].

Few studies address the effects of inhibition of nitric oxide on fetal development. Most of the work on this subject is from the 1990s. In pregnant rats, this nitric oxide synthesis inhibitor causes fetal growth restriction by a reduction in cellular proliferation due to induction of apoptosis [32], reducing the body weight and causing hemorrhagic necrosis of neonate's hind limbs [33, 34].

This suggests that L-NAME crosses the placental barrier and affects the fetal NO synthesis, leading to cell death in the limbs because the NO has a role in limb and digit developments [35]. Reactive oxygen species (ROS) formation by L-NAME induces hemorrhages, oxidative stress, and limb reduction defects [30].

The administration of L-arginine, the precursor of nitric oxide, in mice during gestation promoted an increase in fetal weight presumably due to the contribution of NO in improving fetal-maternal circulation by vasodilation and subsequently increased blood volume and viscosity in the fetal-maternal circulation [36].

4. Effects of inhibition of nitric oxide on fetal heart development in animal models

The first studies on the importance of nitric oxide in cardiac development go back to the beginning of the year 2000. The role of nitric oxide on fetal cardiovascular development is only partially known. In addition, in women who had preeclampsia, their children are at greater risk of developing cardiovascular disease later in life [37].

The nitric oxide probably contributes to the transformation of the epithelium-mesenchyme in the areas of the endocardial cushion, myocardial survival and angiogenesis, and myocardial remodeling. Impaired production of NO in the heart leads to structural congenital abnormalities, resulting in heart failure and increased mortality [38].

Inhibition of nitric oxide during cardiac development is known to promote bicuspid aortic valve defects [39], congenital septal defects, and increase in cardiomyocyte apoptosis [40].

Apoptosis occurs in situations of cardiac remodeling during or after pathological processes and was observed in the myocardium of newborns from rats with hypertension induced by L-NAME. Thus, apoptosis can also occur in postnatal maturation of the heart and other tissues of the cardiovascular system, which need to adapt to the new hemodynamic role [41].

In newborns from L-NAME mothers, the most significant change in the myocardium involved the microvasculature. The wall/lumen ratio of arterioles was significantly higher in neonates of L-NAME and spontaneously hypertensive rats (SHR) than of normotensive mothers at 2 and 15 days postnatal [42].

It is possible that the myocardial vascular changes induced by the blockade of nitric oxide synthesis in rats are due to the activation of the local angiotensin

I-converting enzyme (ACE). Takemoto et al. [43] found an increase in ACE in the coronary arteries and increase of the wall/lumen ratio in the myocardial vasculature of adult rats treated with L-NAME.

A decreased NO generation induces the synthesis of growth-promoting factors from the endothelium. The ACE activation would increase the formation of angiotensin II, which in turn directly induces vascular smooth muscle proliferation [44].

Possibly, the factors involved in hyperplasia/hypertrophy of the smooth muscle cells of the microvasculature of newborns born to hypertensive mothers who received L-NAME during pregnancy are activation of the renin-angiotensin system and activation of the sympathetic nervous system that contributes to the remodeling of intramyocardial vessels [42].

In rats treated with L-NAME, the blood pressure increases via the renin-angiotensin system, and, therefore, angiotensin II can promote the narrowing of the lumen of the microvasculature [45].

In neonates of hypertensive rats induced by L-NAME, in addition to cardiac microvasculature being affected, the pyloric musculature is also compromised, observing hypertrophy and hyperplasia of smooth muscle cells [46].

The rat offspring from L-NAME parents, with sustained NO-induced hypertension, had a remarkably higher blood pressure [47]. In addition to impairment in cardiovascular development, there are other damages in the offspring of rats treated with L-NAME as in the hippocampus, affecting cognitive and learning abilities [48].

5. Effects of inhibition of nitric oxide on fetal renal developmental in animal models

The fetal kidney appears to be extremely vulnerable to the effects of growth retardation. Studies on human infants with growth retardation indicate that the kidneys are disproportionately affected relative to other organs [49].

One study noted that maternal hypertension during pregnancy results in reduced birth weight and a decreased area and number of glomeruli [50]. Certainly, there is a link between maternal environmental factors, particularly nitric oxide inhibition, and the development of hypertension in adulthood.

Some models of arterial hypertension have been studied in animals in order to detect imbalances in fetal development, including protein restriction, excessive sodium intake, impaired uterine or placental circulation, blockade of the renin-angiotensin system (RAS), and increased exposure to maternal glucocorticoids, all of them leading to hypertension in offspring [51–54].

Experimental studies indicate that fetal exposure to an adverse maternal environment may reduce glomerular filtration rate by decreasing the surface area of the glomerular capillaries. In addition, fetal responses to environmental insults, such as maternal hypertension, may contribute to the development of hypertension early in life, including increased expression of apical or basolateral tubular Na^+ carriers and increased production of renal superoxide leading to reabsorption which increased Na^+ [55].

Reductions in NO synthesis decrease renal sodium excretory function, not only through direct action on the renal vasculature but also through modulation of other vasoconstrictor processes and through direct and indirect alterations in tubular sodium transport [56].

Moreover, environmental factors of intrauterine life may worsen the prognosis of offspring hypertension, at least in part, by determining the number of nephrons. The reduced number and size of nephrons may also predispose the individual to the development of progressive renal disease [54, 57].

Kidneys with lower numbers of nephrons maintain their hemodynamic and excretory functions by increasing local vascular resistance and glomerular pressure. The increase in glomerular pressure within the nephrons can trigger a cascade leading to progressive deterioration and loss of nephrons [56].

Nitric oxide is produced within the kidney and plays an important role in the control of many intrarenal processes. NO contributes to the regulation of sodium excretion and thus maintenance of vascular volume and arterial pressure in the adult [50]. Studies have shown that certain animal models of genetic hypertension and forms of human hypertension are associated with a decrease in NO synthesis [58].

The deficient production of NO in the intrauterine period is associated with a reduction in the mass and number of nephrons in the initial period of life. NO is involved in maturation and renal function in the postnatal period [50].

Inhibition of NO synthesis during gestation in rats treated with L-NAME promoted structural changes of the renal microvessels (thickening of the media) in newborns. The remodeling of the microvasculature of the kidneys of the newborns can be involved with adaptive responses to maternal arterial hypertension, activation of local/systemic of RAS in newborns, and enhanced synthesis of peptide growth factors, such as platelet-derived growth factor, which promote smooth muscle cell hyperplasia of the microvasculature [59–61].

Spontaneously hypertensive rats (SHR) at 2 days of age also showed an increase in the area and in the media/lumen ratio of the renal microvasculature due to hypertrophy or hyperplasia of the media layer. Hypertrophy and polyploidy are preferentially found in conduit arterioles, whereas hyperplasia and remodeling are found mainly in small arteries and arterioles [62].

Pups of spontaneously hypertensive rats (SHR) had significantly higher concentrations of renin than Wistar-Kyoto pups from birth until the beginning of the third postnatal week [63] as well as increased expression of angiotensinogen mRNA [64].

The elevated renin concentration of the SHR is linked to increased renal vascular resistance and thus to a reduced renal blood flow and glomerular filtration rate [65]. Also, it appears that sustained activity of the renin-angiotensin system may be required for exaggerated vascular growth responses in SHR [66].

Intrauterine growth restriction by nitric oxide inhibition during pregnancy is associated with a decrease in the number and size glomeruli and microvascular remodeling. Therefore, the nitric oxide inhibition during pregnancy may be linked to structural changes in the kidney which potentially lead to hypertension in later life [54].

Therefore, individuals born after intrauterine growth restriction, such as the L-NAME-induced hypertension model in rats, are at increased risk for kidney and heart morbidities. Endothelial dysfunction, with inhibition of NO synthesis, increases oxidative stress, dysfunction of endothelial progenitor cells, and accelerated vascular aging. L-arginine supplementation and treatment with NO modulators represent promising strategies to improve endothelial function and mitigate long-term outcomes and possibly vascular problems in newborns that have undergone growth restriction during maternal hypertension [67].

6. Conclusions

The inhibition of nitric oxide synthesis during pregnancy promotes changes in the renal and cardiac microvasculature and, in addition, reduction in the number of fetal nephrons, leading to hypertension in the adult life of rat pups and, potentially, in humans. In this sense, the effects of preeclampsia for the mother and the fetus should be considered.

Acknowledgements

The authors are grateful to the National Education Development Fund (FNDE) of the Ministry of Education and Culture (MEC), Brazil, for funding the study.

Conflict of interest

The authors declare no conflict of interest.

Author details

Sonia Jurado[1]*, Kaelly Saraiva[2], Cauane Marceliano[3], Vanessa Souza[3] and Izabela Vieira[3]

1 Associate Professor in Nursing Undergraduate Course, Federal University of Mato Grosso do Sul, Três Lagoas, Brazil

2 Adjunct Professor in Medical Undergraduate Course, Federal University of Mato Grosso do Sul, Três Lagoas, Brazil

3 Nursing Tutorial Education Program (PET), Federal University of Mato Grosso do Sul, Três Lagoas, Brazil

*Address all correspondence to: srjurado@bol.com.br

References

[1] Hodžić J, Izetbegović S, Muračević B, Iriškić R, Jović HS. Nitric oxide biosynthesis during normal pregnancy and pregnancy complicated by preeclampsia. Medicinski Glasnik (Zenica). 2017;**14**(2):211-217. DOI: 10.17392/915-17

[2] Zhao Y, Vanhoutte PM, Leung SWS. Vascular nitric oxide: Beyond eNOS. Journal of Pharmacological Sciences. 2015;**129**:83-94. DOI: 10.1016/j.jphs.2015.09.002

[3] Soma-Pillay P, Nelson-Piercy C, Tolppanen H, Mebazaa A. Physiological changes in pregnancy. Cardiovascular Journal of Africa. 2016;**27**(2):89-84. DOI: 10.5830/CVJA-2016-021

[4] Rachel A, Pakyanadhan S, Abraham S. Impact of l-arginine on nitric oxide regulation in pregnant women prone to preeclampsia: Original research. International Journal of Contemporary Medical Research. 2018;**5**(10):17-21. DOI: 10.21276/ijcmr.2018.5.10.31

[5] Darkwa EO, Djagbletey R, Sottie D, Owoo C, Vanderpuye NM, Essuman R, et al. Serum nitric oxide levels in healthy pregnant women: A case- control study in a tertiary facility in Ghana. Maternal Health, Neonatology and Perinatology. 2018;**4**(3):1-5. DOI: 10.1186/s40748-017-0072-y

[6] Phipps E, Prasanna D, Brima W, Jim B. Preeclampsia: Updates in pathogenesis, definitions, and guidelines. Clinical Journal of the American Society of Nephrology. 2016;**11**(6):1102-1113. DOI: 10.2215/CJN.12081115

[7] Osol G, Barron C, Gokina N, Mandala M. Inhibition of nitric oxide synthases abrogates pregnancy induced uterine vascular expansive remodeling. Journal of Vascular Research. 2009;**46**(5):478-486. DOI: 10.1159/000200963

[8] Spracklen CN, Ryckman KK, Triche EW, Saftlas AF. Physical activity during pregnancy and subsequent risk of preeclampsia and gestational hypertension: A case control study. Maternal and Child Health Journal. 2016;**20**(6):1193-1202. DOI: 10.1007/s10995-016-1919-y

[9] Oliveira CA, Brito HL Jr, Bastos MG, Oliveira FG, Casali TG, Bignoto TC, et al. Depressed cardiac autonomic modulation in patients with chronic kidney disease. Jornal Brasileiro de Nefrologia. 2014;**36**(2):155-162. DOI: 10.5935/0101-2800.20140025

[10] Possomato-Vieira JS, Khalil RA. Mechanisms of endothelial dysfunction in hypertensive pregnancy and preeclampsia. Advances in Pharmacology. 2016;**77**:361-431. DOI: 10.1016/bs.apha.2016.04.008

[11] Dusse LMSA, Vieira LM, Carvalho MG. Hemostatic changes revision in preeclampsia. Jornal Brasileiro de Patologia e Medicina Laboratorial. 2001;**37**(4):267-272. DOI: 10.1590/S1676-24442001000400008

[12] Cavalli RC, Sandrim VC, Santos JET, Duart G. Preeclampsia prediction. Revista Brasileira de Ginecologia e Obstetrícia. 2009;**31**(1):1-4. DOI: 10.1590/S0100-72032009000100001

[13] Su JB. Vascular endothelial dysfunction and pharmacological treatment. World Journal of Cardiology. 2015;**26**:719-741. DOI: 10.4330/wjc.v7.i11.719

[14] Nott A, Riccio A. Nitric oxide-mediated epigenetic mechanisms in developing neurons. Cell Cycle. 2009;**8**:725-730. DOI: 10.4161/cc.8.5.7805

[15] Suzuki T, Mori C, Yoshikawa H, Miyazaki Y, Kansaku N, Tanaka K, et al. Changes in nitric oxide

production levels and expression of nitric oxide synthase isoforms in the rat uterus during pregnancy. Bioscience, Biotechnology, and Biochemistry. 2009;**73**:2163-2166. Available in: https://www.jstage.jst.go.jp/article/bbb/73/10/73_90222/_article

[16] Sprague B, Chesler NC, Magness RR.Shear stress regulation of nitric oxide production in uterine and placental artery endothelial cells: Experimental studies and hemodynamic models of shear stress forces on endothelial cells. The International Journal of Developmental Biology. 2010;**54**(2-3):331-339. DOI: 10.1387/ijdb.082832bs

[17] Rytlewski K, Olszanecki R, Korbut R, Zdebski Z. Effects of prolonged oral supplementation with L-Arginine on blood pressure and nitric oxide synthesis in preeclampsia. European Journal of Clinical Investigation. 2005;**35**(1):32-37. DOI: 10.1111/j.1365-2362.2005.01445

[18] Baban RS. Oxidative stress in recurrent pregnancy loss women. Saudi Medical Journal. 2010;**31**(7):759-763. Available in: http://www.academia.edu/1287698/Oxidative_stress_in_recurrent_pregnancy_loss_women

[19] Meiyappan K, Dhiman P, Rajendiren S, Thayagarajan K, Raghavan SS. Serum nitric oxide and homocysteine as biomarkers of ectopic pregnancy. International Journal of Reproduction, Contraception, Obstetrics and Gynecology. 2015;**4**(1):66-70. DOI: 10.5455/2320-1770.ijrcog20150213

[20] Uzan J, Carbonnel M, Picconne O, Asmar R, Ayoubi J-M. Pre-eclampsia: Pathophysiology, diagnosis, and management. Vascular Health and Risk Management. 2011;**7**:467-474. DOI: 10.2147/VHRM.S20181

[21] Sen S, Rao R, Chaudhuri G. Endothelial cell function in utero-placental circulation physiology and pathophysiology. Current Vascular Pharmacology. 2013;**11**(5):730-736. DOI: 10.2174/1570161111311050010

[22] Krause BJ, Hanson MA, Casanello P. Role of nitric oxide in placental vascular development and function. Placenta. 2011;**32**:797-805. DOI: 10.1016/j.placenta.2011.06.025

[23] Maynard SE, Venkatesha S, Thadhani R, Karumanchi SA. Soluble Fms-like tyrosine kinase 1 and endothelial dysfunction in the pathogenesis of preeclampsia. Pediatric Research. 2005;**57**:1-7. DOI: 10.1203/01.PDR.0000159567.85157.B7

[24] Amraoui F, Spijkers L, Lahsinoui HH, Vogt L, Post JVD, et al. Sflt-1 elevates blood pressure by augmenting endothelin-1-mediated vasoconstriction in mice. PLoS One. 2014;**9**(3):e91897. DOI: 10.1371/journal.pone.0091897

[25] Ziganshina MM, Yarotskaya EL, Bovin NV, Sukhikh GT. Endothelial dysfunction as a consequence of endothelial glycocalyx damage: A role in the pathogenesis of preeclampsia, endothelial dysfunction. In: Lenasi H, editor. Endothelial Dysfunction. England: IntechOpen; 2018. Available in: https://www.intechopen.com/books/endothelial-dysfunction-old-concepts-and-new-challenges/endothelial-dysfunction-as-a-consequence-of-endothelial-glycocalyx-damage-a-role-in-the-pathogenesis

[26] Shu W, Li H, Gong H, Zhang M, Niu X, Yongqiang MA, et al. Evaluation of blood vessel injury, oxidative stress and circulating inflammatory factors in an L-NAME-induced preeclampsia-like rat model. Experimental and Therapeutic Medicine. 2018;**16**:585-594. DOI: 10.3892/etm.2018.6217

[27] Hale SA, Weger L, Mandala M, Osol G. Reduced NO signaling during pregnancy attenuates outward uterine

artery remodeling by altering MMP expression and collagen and elastin deposition. American Journal of Physiology. Heart and Circulatory Physiology. 2011;**301**(4):H1266-H1275. DOI: 10.1152/ajpheart.00519.2011

[28] Araujo AJS, Santos ACV, Souza KS, Aires MB, Santana-Filho VJ, Fioretto ET, et al. Resistance training controls arterial blood pressure in rats with l-name- induced hypertension. Arquivos Brasileiros de Cardiologia. 2013;**100**(4):339-346. DOI: 10.5935/abc.20130051

[29] Leong XF, Ng CY, Jaarin K. Animal models in cardiovascular research: Hypertension and atherosclerosis. BioMed Research International. 2015;**52875**:1-11. DOI: 10.1155/2015/528757

[30] Talebianpoor MS, Delaviz H, Rafei R, Mohammadi B, Sadeghi H, Mohammadi J, et al. Resveratrol attenuates fetal limb malformation and cardiac hypertrophy after preeclampsia induced by L-NAME in pregnant rats. Journal of Pharmaceutical Sciences and Research. 2018;**10**(2):361-364. Available in: https://www.jpsr.pharmainfo.in/Documents/Volumes/vol10Issue02/jpsr10021831.pdf

[31] Cushen SC, Goulopoulou S. New models of pregnancy-associated hypertension. American Journal of Hypertension. 2017;**11**(91):1053-1062. DOI: 10.1093/ajh/hpx063

[32] Miller MJS, Voelker CA, Olister S, Thompson JH, Zhang XJ, Rivera D. Fetal growth retardation in rats may result from apoptosis: Role of peroxynitrite. Free Radical Biology & Medicine. 1996;**21**:619-629. DOI: 10.1016/0891-5849(96)00171-2

[33] Diket AL, Pierce MR, Upender KM, Voelker SS, Eloby-Childress S, Greenberg SS, et al. Nitric oxide inhibition causes intrauterine growth retardation and hind-limb disruptions in rats. American Journal of Obstetrics and Gynecology. 1994;**171**:1243-1250. DOI: 10.1016/0891-5849(96)00171-2

[34] Pierce LR, Pierce MR, Liu H, Kadowitz PJ, Miller MJS. Limb reduction defects after prenatal inhibition of nitric oxide synthase in rats. Pediatric Research. 1996;**38**:905-911. DOI: 10.1203/00006450-199512000-00013

[35] Gregg AR, Schauer A, Shi O, Liu Z, Lee CGL, O'Brien WE. Limb reduction defects in endothelial nitric oxide synthase-deficient mice. American Journal of Physiology. Heart and Circulatory Physiology. 1998;**275**:2319-2324. DOI: 10.1152/ajpheart.1998.275.6.H2319

[36] Al-Bayati MA, Ahmad MA, Khamas W. The potential effect of L-arginine on mice placenta. Advances in Pharmacoepidemiology & Drug Safety. 2014;**3**(2):1-9. DOI: 10.4172/2167-1052.1000150

[37] Davis EF, Lazdam M, Lewandowski AJ, Worton SA, Kelly B, Kenworthy Y, et al. Cardiovascular risk factors in children and young adults born to preeclamptic pregnancies: A systematic review. Pediatrics. 2012;**129**:1552-1561. DOI: 10.1542/peds.2011-3093

[38] Nath AK, Madri JA. The roles of nitric oxide in murine cardiovascular development. Developmental Biology. 2006;**292**:25-33. DOI: 10.1016/j.ydbio.2005.12.039

[39] Lee TC, Zhao YD, Courtman DW, Stewart DJ. Abnormal aortic valve development in mice lacking endothelial nitric oxide synthase. Circulation. 2000;**101**:2345-2348. Available in: https://www.researchgate.net/publication/299010706_Abnormal_aortic_valve_development_in_mice_lacking_endothelial_nitric_oxide_synthase

[40] Feng Q, Song W, Lu X, Hamilton JA, Lei ML, Peng T, et al. Development of heart failure and congenital septal defects in mice lacking endothelial nitric oxide. Circulation. 2000;**106**:873-879. DOI: 10.1161/01.CIR.0000024114.82981.EA

[41] Moreau P, Tea BS, Dam TV, Hamet P. Altered balance between cell replication and apoptosis in hearts and kidneys of newborn SHR. Hypertension. 1997;**30**:720-724. DOI: 10.1161/01.HYP.30.3.720

[42] Jurado SR, Franco RJS, Bankoff ADP, Sanchez A. The heart is a target organ in offspring rats due to maternal hypertension. Journal of Clinical Trials in Cardiology. 2014;**1**(1):1-8. DOI: 10.15226/2374-6882/1/1/00101

[43] Takemoto M, Egashira K, Usui M, Numaguchi K, Tomita H, Tsutsui H, et al. Important role of tissue angiotensin-converting enzyme activity in the pathogenesis of coronary vascular and myocardial structural changes induced by long-term blockade of nitric oxide synthesis in rats. The Journal of Clinical Investigation. 1997;**99**:278-287. DOI: 10.1172/JCI119156

[44] Itoh H, Mukoyama M, Pratt RE, Gibbons GH, Dzau VJ. Multiple autocrine growth factors modulate vascular smooth muscle cell growth response to angiotensin II. The Journal of Clinical Investigation. 1993;**91**: 2268-2274. DOI: 10.1172/JCI116454

[45] Jaarin K, Kamarul ZYN, Qodriyah HMS, Azman A, Zuhair JSF, Juliana AH, et al. Mechanisms of the antihypertensive effects of *Nigella sativa* oil in L-NAME-induced hypertensive rats. Clinics (São Paulo). 2015;**70**(11):751-757. DOI: 10.6061/clinics/2015(11)07

[46] Voelker CA, Miller MJS, Zhang XJ, Childress E, Clark DA, Pierce MR. Perinatal nitric oxide synthase inhibition retards neonatal growth by inducing hypertrophic pyloric stenosis in rats. Pediatric Research. 1995;**38**:768-774. DOI: 10.1203/00006450-199511000-00022

[47] Gerová M, Bernátová I, Török J, Jurani M. Cardiovascular system in offsprings of hypertensive rats with defective nitric oxide production. Physiological Research. 2002;**51**:465-474. Available in: http://www.biomed.cas.cz/physiolres/pdf/51/51_465.pdf

[48] Zhu H, Zhu W, Hu R, Wang H, Ma D, Li X. The effect of pre-eclampsia-like syndrome induced by L-NAME on learning and memory and hippocampal glucocorticoid receptor expression: A rat model. Hypertension in Pregnancy. 2017;**36**(1):36-43. DOI: 10.1080/10641955.2016.1228957

[49] Wintour EM, Johnson K, Koukoulas I, Moritz K, Tersteeg M, Dodic M. Programming the cardiovascular system, kidney and the brain—A review. Placenta. 2003;**24**: 65-71. DOI: 10.1053/plac.2002.0927

[50] Singh RR, Easton LK, Booth LC, Schlaich MP, Head GA, Moritz KM, et al. Renal nitric oxide deficiency and chronic kidney disease in young sheep born with a solitary functioning kidney. Scientific Reports. 2017;**6**:26777. DOI: 10.1038/srep26777

[51] Woods LL, Ingelfinger JR, Nyengaard JR, Rasch R. Maternal protein restriction suppresses the newborn renin-angiotensin system and programs adult hypertension in rats. Pediatric Research. 2001;**49**:460-467. Available in: https://www.nature.com/articles/pr200173

[52] Langley-Evans SC. Fetal programming of cardiovascular function through exposure to maternal undernutrition. The Proceedings of the Nutrition Society. 2001;**60**:505-513. DOI: 10.1079/PNS2001111

[53] Woods LL, Rasch R. Perinatal Ang II programs adult blood pressure, glomerular number, and renal function in rats. The American Journal of Physiology. 1998;**275**:1593-1599. DOI: 10.1152/ajpregu.1998.275.5.R1593

[54] Solhaug MJ, Dong XQ, Adelman RD, Dong KW. Ontogeny of neuronal nitric oxide synthase, NOSI, in the developing porcine kidney. American Journal of Physiology. Regulatory, Integrative and Comparative Physiology. 2000;**278**:1453-1459. DOI: 10.1152/ajpregu.2000.278.6.R1453

[55] Paixão AD, Alexander BT. How the kidney is impacted by the perinatal maternal environment to develop hypertension. Biology of Reproduction. 2013;**89**(6):1-10. DOI: 10.1095/biolreprod.113.111823

[56] Schnackenberg C, Patel AR, Kirchner KA, Granger JP. Nitric oxide, the kidney and hypertension. Clinical and Experimental Pharmacology & Physiology. 1997;**24**:600-606. DOI: 10.1111/j.1440-1681.1997.tb02099.x

[57] The Low Birth Weight and Nephron Number Working Group. The impact of kidney development on the life course: A consensus document for action. Nephron. 2017;**136**(1):3-49. DOI: 10.1159/000457967

[58] Tain YL, Hsieh CS, Lin IC, Chen CC, Shen JM, Huang LT. Effects of maternal L-citrulline supplementation on renal function and blood pressure in offspring exposed to maternal caloric restriction: The impact of nitric oxide pathway. Nitric Oxide. 2010;**23**(1):34-41. DOI: 10.1016/j.niox.2010.03.005

[59] Jurado SR. Effects of the maternal hypertension in renal development in offspring of rats. Journal of Clinical & Experimental Cardiology. 2014;**5**(4):1-5. DOI: 10.4172/2155-9880.1000306

[60] Kourembanas S, McQuillan LP, Leung GK, Faller DV. Nitric oxide regulates the expression of vasoconstrictors and growth factors by vascular endothelium under normoxia and hypoxia. The Journal of Clinical Investigation. 1993;**92**:99-104. DOI: 10.1172/JCI116604

[61] Numaguchi K, Egashira K, Takemoto M, Kadokami T, Shimokawa H, Sueishi K, et al. Chronic inhibition of nitric oxide synthesis causes coronary microvascular remodeling in rats. Hypertension. 1995;**26**:957-962. Available in: https://www.ncbi.nlm.nih.gov/pubmed/7490155

[62] Bravo R, Somoza B, Ruiz-Gayo M, González C, Ruilope LM, Fernández-Alfonso MS. Differential effect of chronic antihypertensive treatment on vascular smooth muscle cell phenotype in spontaneously hypertensive rats. Hypertension. 2001;**37**:4-10. DOI: 10.1161/01.HYP.37.5.e4

[63] Sinaiko A, Mirkin BL. Ontogenesis of the renin-angiotensin system in spontaneously hypertensive and normotensive Wistar rats. Circulation Research. 1974;**34**:693-696. DOI: 10.1161/01.res.34.5.693

[64] Gomez RA, Lynch KR, Chevalier RL, Wilfong N, Everett A, Carey RM, et al. Renin and angiotensinogen gene expression in maturing rat kidney. The American Journal of Physiology. 1988;**254**:582-587. DOI: 10.1152/ajprenal.1988.254.4.F582

[65] Harrap SB, Nicolaci J, Doyle AE. Persistent effects on blood pressure and renal hemodynamics following chronic converting enzyme inhibition with perindopril. Clinical and Experimental Pharmacology & Physiology. 1986;**13**:753-765. DOI: 10.1111/j.1440-1681.1986.tb02379.x

[66] Black MJ, Niklaus A, Bertram JF, Diley R, Alex B. Vascular growth

responses in SHR and WKY during development of renal (1K1C). American Journal of Hypertension. 1997;**10**(1):43-50. DOI: 10.1016/S0895-7061(96)00255-5

[67] Yzydorzyk C, Armengaud J, Peyter A, Chehade H, Cachat F, Juvet C, et al. Endothelial dysfunction in individuals born after fetal growth restriction: Cardiovascular and renal consequences and preventive. Journal of Developmental Origins of Health and Disease. 2017;**8**(4):448-464. DOI: 10.1017/S2040174417000265

Chapter 7

Alloimmunization and Role of HLA in Pregnancy

Meenakshi Singh, Jyoti Rajak, Shalaka Kadam and Sunil B. Rajadhyaksha

Abstract

Alloimmunization also known as isoimmunization, during pregnancy is the production of IgG antibodies by the mother against the paternally inherited antigens (IPA) in the foetus/newborn. The alloimmunization during pregnancy leads to various alloimmune disorders, such as, haemolytic disease of the foetus and newborn (HDFN), neonatal alloimmune neutropenia (NAN) and foetal and neonatal alloimmune thrombocytopenia (FNAIT) due to the production of maternal alloantibodies against the red blood cell antigen, neutrophils and platelets cell antigens, respectively. Recent studies suggest that maternal anti-HLA class I alloantibodies may also be the cause of FNAIT in addition to antibodies against platelet antigens. On the contrary, studies have also suggested that HLA-C, a classical HLA class I molecule, and HLA-G, a nonclassical HLA molecule, play an important role in placentation and modulation of the maternal immune system during pregnancy, respectively, and thereby leading to acceptance of the semi allogeneic fetus. So far most of the studies have discussed alloimmunization in pregnancy relating to Rh antigen. Thus, in this chapter an attempt has been made to discuss alloimmunization in pregnancy caused because of maternal alloantibody against HLA antigen and its role in immune modulation during pregnancy.

Keywords: HLA, MHC, HLA-G, IPA

1. Introduction

Mammalian pregnancy with haemochorial placentation is an immunological contradiction with suppression of an immune response against the semi allogeneic foetus having inherited paternal antigens foreign to mother [1]. The foetus is not rejected as it would have, ideally in case of an unmatched organ transplant, wherein the immune system forbids the incursion of any genetic material or protein foreign to itself [2].

The protective mechanism which leads to acceptance of the semi allogeneic foetus includes: (i) Complete separation of maternal and foetal blood circulation. (ii) Low expression of foetal antigens that may stimulate graft rejection. The trophoblast cells originating from foetus lack expression of classical HLA class Ia and class II antigen except for very low expression of HLA-C antigens. They express HLA class Ib antigens which are known to modulate immune responses at the feto-maternal interface [3]. (iii) Involvement of both mother and foetus in order to maintain pregnant uterus as an immune privileged site. (iv) Programming of the maternal immune response by factors obtained from placental and extra placental membrane [4].

Maternal and foetal cells interact in co-ordination to maintain an immune privileged environment at feto-maternal interface; some instances do occur which lead to maternal sensitization thereby leading to various disorders in the foetus/neonate. Alloimmunization during pregnancy is the stimulation of maternal immune response by the paternal inherited foetal or placental antigens [5].

The recognition of antigens as self and non-self is the essential process by which the immune system determines whether or not to develop an immune response. The response of the maternal immune system will depend on genetic and acquired factors related to the foetus and to antigen immunogenicity. Maternal alloimmunization occurs when the foetal and the maternal lymph combine due to rupture of placental barrier which often happens during delivery, although feto-maternal haemorrhage (FMH) may also result early in pregnancy. The instance of FMH has been observed in 7, 16, and 29% of mothers during their first, second and third trimesters, respectively [6]. Other maternal factors responsible for maternal sensitization involve factors such as Rh incompatibility, major surgical procedure, blood transfusion, multiparity, or operative removal of placenta [7].

The major antigens against which the maternal alloimmunization occurs are RBC, granulocytes (neutrophils), human platelet antigens and HLA antigens. The sensitization against these antigens leads to disorders, such as, haemolytic disease of foetus and newborn (HDFN), neonatal alloimmune neutropenia (NAN) and foetal and neonatal alloimmune thrombocytopenia (FNAIT), respectively.

Till now most of the studies have addressed the maternal alloimmunization relating to Rh and platelet antigen, this book chapter aims at exploring the role of human leukocyte antigen (HLA) in pregnancy and alloimmunization along with other factors.

2. Role of HLA in pregnancy

The human leukocyte antigen (HLA) also known as the major histocompatibility complex (MHC) play a very crucial role in enabling the immune system to differentiate between "self" and "non-self-antigen" [8]. It is situated on the short arm of human chromosome 6p21.3, and codes for nearly 130 structural genes known to function in antigen presentation to immune system thereby modulating the immune response. It is categorized into three classes i.e., class I, class II and class III [9]. The HLA class I gene is further classified into classical HLA class Ia genes (HLA-A, -B, -C) and non-classical HLA class Ib genes (HLA-E, -F, -G) [3]. The non-classical HLA class Ib genes show limited polymorphism as compared to those of classical HLA class Ia genes [10]. The HLA class II is differentiated into HLA-DR,-DQ,-DM and -DP.

The HLA class I molecules are known to interact with CD8+ T cells, natural killer cells (NK cells), and class II molecules with CD4+ T cells, respectively [11, 12] to elicit an immune response in order to eliminate the foreign or non-self-antigens. In contrast the non-classical HLA class Ib molecules interact with natural killer cells (NK cells) and other immune cell to develop an immunological tolerogenic effect. HLA plays a very important role in transplantation, as it is known to evoke an immune response to the transplanted graft, thus are very critical in pregnancy from gamete formation to completion of development, as foetus is the most successful semi-allograft.

The non-classical HLA class Ib molecules, primarily HLA-G plays a very important role in maintaining maternal tolerance i.e., an immunosuppressive state during pregnancy thereby contributing to foetal endurance and growth. Consequently inability in maintaining the maternal tolerance to the foetus, adversely affects the pregnancy leading to complications such as recurrent spontaneous abortion, foetal growth restriction, and preeclampsia [13]. Also HLA-C along with KIR (killer-immunoglobulin receptor) has been implicated to play a role in placentation. Thus, the role of HLA along with other immune cells may be implicated in maintaining pregnancy as well as at time in leading to pregnancy complications.

2.1 HLA-G in immune modulation during pregnancy

Among the non-classical HLA class Ib genes HLA-G is the most studied because of its role in immune modulation during pregnancy and its association with complexities like pre-eclampsia and recurrent spontaneous abortion in pregnancy [14].

2.1.1 Structure and expression of HLA-G

The non-classical class Ib HLA-G gene is situated near to the classical class Ia HLA-A gene on chromosome 6 and is also greatly homologous to it. The HLA-G gene comprises of seven intronic regions and eight exonic regions. The exon 1 codes for the signal peptide. The exons 2–4 code for the external part of HLA-G molecule which consist of three parts viz. α1, α2 and α3 domains, exon 5 encodes for the transmembrane region, where as exon 6 and a very short part of exon 8 encode for the cytoplasmic tail of the HLA-G molecule. The HLA-G gene is translated into a 38 kDa protein having similar structure as that of HLA class I antigens. It consists of a heavy chain that binds a light chain β2-microglobulin a protein coded by a gene on chromosome 15. The α1 and α2 extracellular domain of heavy chain form the peptide binding groove [15].

The HLA-G antigen has seven splice variants (HLA-G1-HLA-G7) as a result of alternative splicing event of the mRNA from the single HLA-G gene, of which HLA-G1 is the full length variant and the rest are formed by out-splicing of exons. Out of the seven isoform HLA-G1, HLA-G2, HLA- G3 and HLA-G4 are membrane-bound and the remaining three i.e., sHLA-G5, sHLA-G6 and sHLA-G7 are soluble isoforms [16]. The coding region of HLA-G gene shows meagre polymorphism but the polymorphisms that are present are equally shared by introns and exon 2, 3 and 4. Most of these polymorphism do not modify the protein sequence and those which do modify the protein sequence permit to be grouped in major allele groups like G*01::xx, G*01:02, G*01:03: xx, G*01:04: xx, G*01:05 N (null allele), G*01:06, and G*01:07 to G*01:18. Overall there are 61 alleles and 19 protein groups representing an amino acid substitution have been delineated in the HLA-G gene sequence [WHO Nomenclature Committee for factors of the HLA System and the International Immunogenetics Information System (IMGT)/HLA Database] [15].

HLA-G expression was first reported on human non-villous cytotrophoblast cells [17]. Its expression is stringently confined to certain cells, being largely expressed in extravillous cytotrophoblast cells. HLA-G5 a soluble variant is present throughout the placenta, within the chorion membrane, maternal blood and the decidua [18]. Apart from placental expression soluble HLA-G proteins are present in peripheral blood of pregnant women, non-pregnant women and men. The presence of sHLA-G in the blood of non-pregnant women indicates that it may play an important role in reproduction even before conception. Soluble HLA-G is also found in follicular fluid, fertilized oocyte and in male reproductive tissue including semen [14]. HLA-G presence can also be detected in tissues like thymic medulla, cornea, pancreas and in human mononuclear phagocytic cells [53]. Its expression can be stimulated in condition following transplant, viral infections, autoimmune diseases and tumors [19].

2.1.2 HLA-G polymorphism

Both coding and non-coding regions of HLA-G gene display polymorphism. Exonic polymorphism may affect biological function such as binding of peptides or production of isoforms; whereas intronic polymorphism may influence the expression of the gene. Codon 31, 35, 57 and 69 of Exon 2 and codon 93, 107 and 110 of exon 3 coding region display majority of the polymorphism. A large number of SNPs (single nucleotide polymorphism) have been found in the non-coding region, including the promoter region at 5′UTR (untranslated region) and the 3′UTR. Some of these polymorphisms located near the regulatory element have an impact on the binding of the corresponding factors.

A 14 bp deletion/insertion have also been reported in the 3′UTR region of exon 8. These 14 bp del/ins are suspected to affect the size and stability of the mRNA transcripts. It was noticed by Rousseau et al. that a 14 bp insertion of sequence (5′-ATTTGTTCATGCCT-3′) lead to deletion of 92 bp sequence in the 3′UTR region, thereby resulting in production of more stable transcript. Few polymorphisms that may also effect the stability of mRNA transcripts, including the SNPs located at the position +3142 (C/G) and at +3172 position (G/A) in the 3′UTR region [19].

2.1.3 Immune modulation by HLA-G during pregnancy

Approximately 40% of the decidual tissue comprise of maternal immune cells at the beginning of pregnancy. Majority of these immune cells are natural killer (CD56 bright 16−) cells which are distinct from the NK cells (CD56 dim16+) present in the peripheral blood as the decidual NK cells have reduced cytotoxic activity. Also the decidual NK cells have a higher expression for genes encoding for integrins, lectin-like receptors, KIR (killer-immunoglobulin like receptors) and cytokines. Along with the presence of NK cell decidual tissue also show the presences of macrophages, T lymphocytes and dendritic cell [19, 20].

The trophoblast cells of the embryo express HLA-G antigen since the beginning of the first trimester and are present till the end of pregnancy. The interaction of HLA-G protein at the feto-maternal interface with the immune cell of the decidua ensures the foetal tolerance by inhibition of cytotoxic activity of NK cells and CD8+ T cells, suppressing the proliferation of alloreactive CD4+ T cells, suppressing the B cell activity, leading to the secretion of Th2 cytokines and stimulation of regulatory T cells (Treg) [19].

HLA-G intercedes its immunosuppressive activity by interaction of alpha 1 domain with inhibitory receptors expressed on immune cells. Leukocytes express inhibitory receptors like immunoglobulin-like transcripts (ILT)-2, ILT-4 and KIR. CD4+ and CD8+ T cells, B cells, monocytes, macrophages and myeloid dendritic cells (DC) display ILT-2, interact with only heterodimers of HLA-G1 or sHLA-G5 and ß2m. ILT-4 displayed by monocytes, macrophages and myeloid DC's have the capability to also interact with monomers of HLA-G whereas the NK cells interact through the KIR2DL4 expressed by them [19] (**Figure 1**). The interaction of these immune cells like decidual NK cells, CD4+ and CD8+ T cells which are

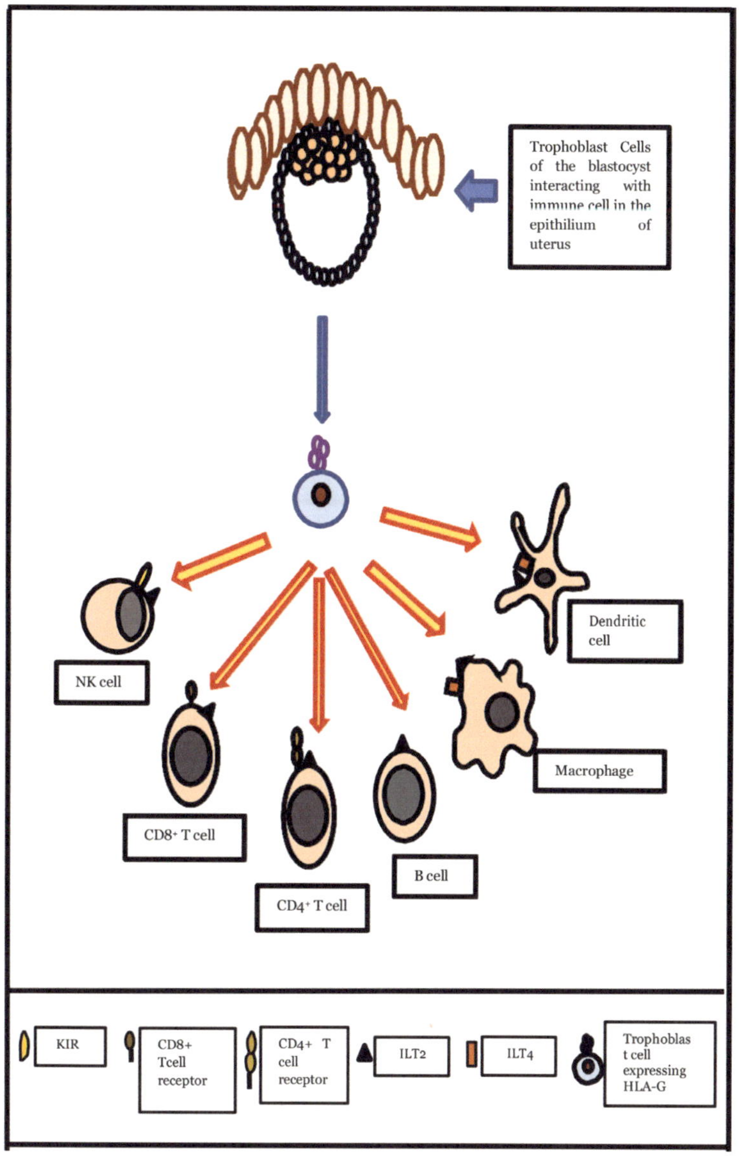

Figure 1.
HLA-G molecules expressed by the trophoblast cells interact with the inhibitory receptor KIR2DL4 expressed by the NK cells, ILT-2 (Ig-like transcript 2) expressed by NK cells, CD4+ and CD8+ T-cells and B-cells, and ILT-2 and ILT-4 expressed by macrophages and dendritic cells. The interaction of the HLA-G with its cognate receptors leads to immune tolerogenic effect thereby leading to the acceptance of the foetus by the maternal immune system.

HLA-G negative cells with trophoblast cell expressing HLA-G molecule leads to the acquisition of HLA-G molecule by immune cells thereby making them HLA-G+ cells through a process called as trogocytosis. Trogocytosis is a mechanism by which surface molecules may be transferred from one cell to another via cell to cell contact. The acquisition of the HLA-G molecule by these immune cells contributes to an immune suppressive milieu without them expressing HLA-G molecule, but only temporarily displaying it [21]. The acquiring of the HLA-G molecule by the decidual NK cells is preceded by a cycle of internalization, degradation and reacquisition of HLA-G. This cycle helps NK cells to maintain both tolerance and immune function [20].

2.1.4 HLA-G and pregnancy disorders

Abnormal placentation and immunological interaction at the feto-maternal interface are believed to play very crucial role in placenta-mediated complication of late pregnancy (viz. pre-eclampsia, foetal growth restriction, still birth and placental abruption) and foetal rejection in some pathological pregnancy, respectively. Deficient level of HLA-G expression and polymorphisms at HLA-G loci are known to be correlated to pregnancy complication especially pre-eclampsia and recurrent miscarriages (RM).

Pre-eclampsia is a pregnancy disorder which is clinically evident in the late second and third trimester of pregnancy [19]. It is characterised by high blood pressure, proteinuria and oedema associated with organ damage and prematurity. It is known to be a major cause of perinatal deaths, premature births and intrauterine growth restriction with an occurrence of 5–10% of all the pregnancy [22]. Though the major cause is unknown, various studies suggest that it may be related to maladapted immune system, with low levels of immune regulatory cell and low expression of HLA-G molecules [23]. The development of pregnancy has been strongly associated with level of soluble HLA-G molecules in the maternal blood. Maternal serum with higher levels of sHLA-G has been identified in females with successful pregnancy when compared with pre-eclampsia patients [24]. Lower sHLA-G levels in the maternal blood, with down regulated HLA-G and decreased proportion of HLA-G+ cells have been identified in patients with preeclampsia and are thought to be are strongly associated with preeclampsia [24–26]. The 14 bp ins/del in the 3′UTR of region exon 8 have been extensively studied, and it has been reported to be related to severe pre-eclampsia [15]. But on the contrary, there are studies which have reported no significant association of the 14 bp polymorphism with preeclampsia [24–26] implicating that differences in the ethnic population should be considered for the association between HLA-G 14 bp polymorphism and serum sHLA-G level. The SNP at position +3172 (G/A) leading to decreased in mRNA stability has been linked to pre-eclampsia [19]. Steinborn et al. reported that women with soluble HLA-G levels lower than 9.95 ng/ml have a risk of 7.1 for developing placental abruption during pregnancy as compared to healthy women [3].

Recurrent spontaneous abortion (RSA) is defined as the loss of two or more consecutive pregnancy with the same partner [27]. The major causes of RSA are considered to be chromosomal abnormalities, anatomical anomalies and endocrine disorders along with immunologic dysfunction [28]. Many studies have reported increased occurrence of HLA-G allele homozygous for 14 bp ins in women with RSA [19]. Also, a study has reported that decreased expression of HLA-G suppresses the function of decidual NK cells and thereby may lead to RSA [28]. SNPs−1573T>C and −1746C>A in the promoter region of HLA-G gene are shown to be associated with RSA [29]. As the level of sHLA-G is known to be associated with the pregnancy complication, the measurement of sHLA-G protein may be useful in primary diagnosis for the pathogenesis of pregnancy complications.

2.2 Role of HLA-C and KIR during pregnancy

Health of a foetus during pregnancy depends on the supply of nutrients and oxygen to the placenta. During placentation the foetal trophoblast cells infiltrate into the uterine wall, transforming the spiral artery (maternal artery supplying blood to the placenta) into a high-conductance vessel, thereby increasing the blood flow to about 100 folds [30]. This transformation allows adequate time for gas exchange and also provides sufficient nourishment to the foetus. Defective infiltration of the trophoblast cells into the uterus leads to failure in arterial conversion, thereby leading the arterial blood to squirt into the intervillous space from the non-transformed arteries causing impairment of the villous tree (placentation). The impaired placentation leads to reduced transport of oxygen and starving of the foetus. The clinical manifestation of this failure may result in disorders such foetal growth restriction (FGR), preeclampsia, recurrent miscarriage (RM), unexplained still birth, placental abruption and preterm labour [31, 32].

The uterus shows abundance of decidual natural killer cells (NK cells) and thus, is thought to be involved in placentation and thereby in foetal development. Placenta is the site at which maternal allorecognition of the foetus takes place, wherein the foetal extra villous trophoblast cells (EVTs) encroach and unify with the maternal immune cells. Interaction of maternal KIR present on the uterine NK cells and its corresponding ligand, HLA-C which is the only classical HLA class I antigen expressed on the trophoblast cells of the foetus are claimed to regulate the process of placentation.

There are approximately 14 different KIR genes existing in a linear array in the leukocyte receptor complex (LRC) on chromosome 19q13.4. KIRs are differentiated on the basis of number of extracellular Ig-like domain (2 or 3) and cytoplasmic tail (long or short). They are known to regulate the activity of NK cells, either conferring them with an inhibitory or activating signal. Interaction of KIR with a long cytoplasmic tail (e.g., KIR2DL1) with its corresponding ligands leads to generation of an inhibitory signal, where as those having a short tail (e.g., KIR2DS1) results in activation of NK cells.

The activating and inhibitory genes are differentiated into two haplotype A and B. The KIR A haplotype is the most frequently occurring haplotype and consists of six inhibitory genes. The KIR B haplotype consist of gene which are more variable in their genetic content and are mostly activating KIR. Hence an individual's KIR genotype can be designated as "AA", "AB", and "BB".

The most important ligand for KIR is the HLA-C molecules, and there are approximately 4000 alleles of HLA-C. The HLA-C are differentiated into two distinct group by KIR, i.e., HLA-C1 and HLA-C2 [33]. HLA-C molecules with amino acid asparagine (Asn) at position 80 belong to HLA-C1 group, where as those with amino acid lysine (Lys) at the 80th position belong to group C2 of HLA-C. KIR2DL2/3 (inhibitory receptor) interacts with HLA-C1 allotype and KIR2DL1 and KIR2DS1 act as receptors for HLA-C present in C2 group [34].

Existence of KIR B haplotype in mother confers protection from pregnancy complications, where as its absence may increase the risk of complications [35]. The KIR B haplotype consist of activating KIR2DS1 receptor, which on interacting with its cognate ligand induces the NK cells to secrete granulocyte-macrophage colony stimulating factors and other chemokines known to promote placental trophoblast invasion. It also consists of KIR2DL1*004 which is the most common inhibitory KIR2DL1 allele on the B haplotype, and is known to have a weak interaction with HLA-C2 allotype as compared to alleles present on KIR A haplotype [36]. On the contrary, mothers homozygous for KIR A haplotypes (KIR "AA" genotype), with foetus having an additional C2 copy as compared to mother (i.e., mother C1/C2 with foetus C1/C2 or mother C1/C2 with foetus C2/C2), that to when the extra copy is of paternal origin are at an increased risk of having a complicated pregnancy [6]. As mothers with KIR AA haplotype have two copies of inherited inhibitory KIR for HLA-C2 allotype i.e., KIR2DL1, thus when the mothers uterine NK cells possessing KIR AA genotype interact with foetal trophoblast cells expressing HLA-C2 allotype, it induces a strong inhibitory effect on NK cell which is one of the reasons for defective placentation and in turn for various pregnancy related complications [37] (**Figure 2**).

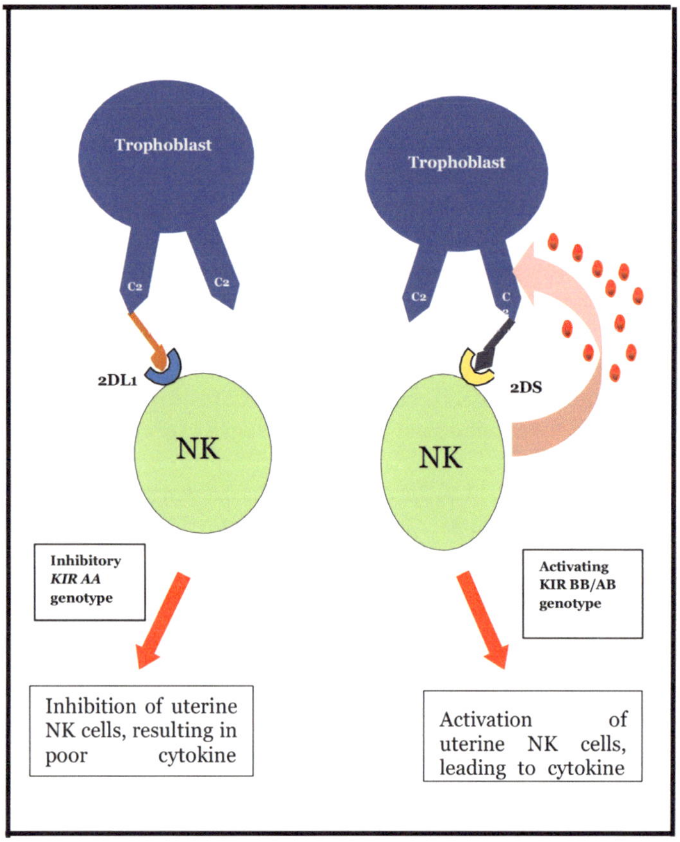

Figure 2.
Model for maternal KIR/foetal HLA-C interaction at the placentation site. The figure depicts foetus homozygous for HLA-C2 group with one paternally inherited HLA-C2 molecule. If the mother possesses KIR AA genotype, then the inhibitory KIR2DL1 receptor will interact with HLA-C2 molecule expressed by trophoblast cells leading to strong inhibition of uterine NK cells thereby resulting in defective placentation. On the contrary if the mother possess KIR AB or BB genotype, the activating KIR2DS1 receptor present in the KIR B haplotype interacts with HLA-C2 molecule expressed by trophoblast cells stimulating the of uterine NK to produce cytokines such as GM-CSF thereby resulting in normal placentation.

2.3 Clinical impact of H-Y alloimmunity in secondary recurrent miscarriages (SRM)

H-Y antigens are a class of minor histocompatibility antigens (mHAs), encoded on Y-chromosome are omnipresent in male cells including foetal and trophoblast cells. H-Y antigens exhibit a large amount of similarity to H-X antigen encoded on the X-chromosome, but they possess few distinct regions which make them highly immunogenic in nature. The H-Y alloimmunity has turned out to be, one of the potential reasons for SRM during pregnancy.

SRM is defined as three or more consecutive miscarriages following a successful pregnancy as compared to primary recurrent miscarriage (PRM), which is characterized by three or more miscarriages without a previous successful birth. PRM is supposed to be caused because of chromosomal defect along with improper implantation of the embryo, whereas SRM are more probably caused due to immunological responses [38].

Generally, during pregnancy the cellular and humoral anti-HY immune response is well tolerated by the foetus, but in minority of cases the H-Y alloimmune response may lead to complications during early or late pregnancy. It has been implicated that pregnancy with a male foetus results in the development of alloimmune response towards the H-Y antigen by mother's immune system, thereby predisposing the mother to SRM and also impacting the prospect of subsequent pregnancy negatively in terms of perinatal complications and live birth [38, 39].

The presence of H-Y restricted HLA alleles along with H-Y antibodies, have also been related to the development of SRM and other pregnancy complications [38, 40]. The term "H-Y restricting HLA" is utilized to describe HLA alleles documented till date, which functionally exhibit H-Y peptides. H-Y restricting HLA alleles include the following HLA class I alleles: HLA-A*01, HLAA*02, HLA-B*07, HLA-B*08, HLA-B*52, HLA-B*60 and HLA class II alleles: HLA-DRB1*15, -DQB1* 0501/2, -DRB3*03.

Possessing a HY restricting HLA class II alleles substantially decreases the prospect of live birth in patients with SRM and firstborn boys as compared to those with firstborn girl. It is implicated that the prospect of live birth decreases in a dose-response fashion with increasing number of maternal HY-restricting HLA class II alleles in patients with firstborn boys [40]. Maternal possession of HY restricting HLA class II alleles also reduces the long-term chance of live birth in females with SRM [41]. Whereas a mother homozygous for HLA-G 14 bps ins and carrying HY restricting class II alleles are predisposed to SRM with the first born boy and also negatively affect the birth weight of the boy [42].

In a study, antibodies against both HLA and H-Y antigens during early pregnancy were significantly higher in SRM females as compared to females with normal pregnancy. The prevalence of these antibodies were associated to low subsequent live birth rate whereas the existence of anti H-Y antibodies were related to low male/female ratio in subsequent live births [40]. The male: female ratio for SRM was observed to be 1.49 prior to miscarriages and 0.76 subsequent to miscarriages in a 20 years cohort study [38]. Thus, implicating H-Y antibodies in preventing implantation or successful gestation of male foetus. Considering H-Y antibodies as one of the factors responsible for SRM, IVIG (intravenous immunoglobulin) infusions are commonly used as treatment to neutralize the circulating antibodies, and it has been shown to improve the birth rates in patients with SRM [38].

3. Rh alloimmunization

The rhesus (Rh) blood group system comprises of more than 50 independent antigens and is highly polymorphic of the human blood group [43]. Following ABO, Rh blood grouping system is clinically important in transfusion medicine. The common Rh antigens are D, C or c, and E or e. Of which the D-antigen is greatly immunogenic and stimulates an immune response in 80% of person negative for D-antigen, when transfused with a D-antigen positive blood [44, 45]. Thus, D-antigen typing is routinely performed on every blood donor and transfusion recipient in order to avoid clinical complications due to mismatched transfusions. On the contrary, even with the use of anti-D immunoglobulin prophylaxis, there is still occurrence of D-alloimmunization in pregnancy.

D-alloimmunization (Rh alloimmunization) in pregnancy occurs due to incompatibility of D-antigen between the mother and the foetus. Generally, an individual is categorized as Rh-positive if they show an expression of Rh D-antigen on the erythrocytes, and Rh negative if there is no expression of D-antigen on the erythrocyte surface [46]. The Rh alloimmunization becomes clinically substantial when an Rh negative mother carries a foetus which is Rh-positive. The incompatibility of Rh antigen leads to sensitization of mother to the D-antigen, and also to the production of anti-D antibodies, which can adhere to and possibly lead to destruction of

Rh-positive erythrocytes of foetus. Nevertheless, the Rh incompatibility typically does not have an adverse consequence on the initial pregnancy as the foetus is delivered prior to the development of anti-D alloimmune response [47]. Although, it may also occur during the initial pregnancy due to spontaneous antenatal mixing of the foetal and maternal blood. In some instances such as miscarriage, abortion, trauma, childbirth and invasive prenatal diagnosis viz. chorionic villous sampling, amniocentesis, and pregnancy related uterine curettage may lead to feto-maternal haemorrhage thereby causing maternal exposure to foetal blood and consequently leading to alloimmunization [48]. The risk of Rh D immunization is estimated to be 1.5–2% in sensitized women following spontaneous miscarriage and 4–5% after dilation and curettage [49, 50]. Once the mother has been alloimmunized, subsequent pregnancies are at an increased risk, for the development of haemolytic disease of the new born (HDN) if the foetus is incompatible i.e., Rh-positive [45]. The diagnostic and clinical management of HDN is described in Section 4.1.

4. Disease caused due to alloimmunization in pregnancy

4.1 Haemolytic disease of foetus/newborn (HDFN)

Alloantibodies against the Rh antigen are the most common reason for intensive haemolytic disease in the neonates. Although the rate at which clinically significant HDFN occurs is relatively low viz. 3/100,000–80/100,000 live births [51]. In comparison to Rh antigen, alloantibodies to Kell (K and k), Duffy (Fya), Kidd (Jka and Jkb), and MNSs (M, N, S, and s) antigens, are also known to lead severe haemolytic disease in the foetus [52]. Although over 50 different non-ABO red cell surface antigens are thought to be involved in leading to HDFN, but the most relevant and significant alloantibodies causing HDFN are anti-RhD [44], anti-Rhc, and anti-Kell (K1) [53]. HDN due to Kell alloimmunization results in haemolysis and direct inhibition of erythropoiesis by Kell antibodies, as the Kell antigen is expressed on the surface of erythroid progenitor [6, 54]. Alloimmunization due to anti-Kell antibodies results in critical foetal disease even at lower maternal antibody titre than in Rhesus disease [6]. ABO incompatibility also causes HDN, but it occurs exclusively in mother with type-O blood with foetus having type-A or type-B blood. 1% of the type-O mothers possess a high titre of IgG antibodies against both A and B antigens. They cross the placental barrier and lead to haemolysis. Mothers with type-A or type-B antigen have the occurrence of IgM antibodies which are incapable of crossing the placental barrier thus have no role in alloimmunization during pregnancy [6].

A neonate delivered by an alloimmunized mother displays clinical indication based on the severity of the disease. General indications are jaundice, pallor, hepatosplenomegaly, and foetal hydrops in severe cases. Neonates with HDN very frequently suffer anaemia due to destruction of RBCs by reticuloendothelial system and in some due to intravascular destruction. Rarely conjugated hyperbilirubinemia is suffered by the neonate due to placental or hepatic dysfunction with severe haemolytic disease.

Foetal anaemia can be diagnosed using ultrasound, cardiotocography and cordocentesis [48]. High resolution ultrasonography has supported in early diagnosis of early hydrops and has also lowered the foetal trauma and fatality rate to approximately 2% while performing percutaneous umbilical blood sampling (PUBS) and placental trauma during amniocentesis. Rh and ABO alloimmunization can be diagnosed using indirect Coombs test and direct antibody test [6]. Currently in order to prevent alloimmunization in mothers having maternal and foetal Rh incompatibility Rh immunoglobulin (RhIG) is administered at the 28th week of pregnancy. This has critically helped in reducing the instances of HDFN due to anti-D alloantibody [6, 55]. Postnatal HDFN treatment consists of intensive phototherapy and exchange transfusions to treat severe hyperbilirubinemia and top-up transfusions to treat early and late anaemia [56].

4.2 Foetal/neonatal alloimmune thrombocytopenia (FNAIT)

Maternal alloantibodies against foetal human platelet antigens (HPA) cause FNAIT. It is comparatively an infrequent condition occurring in 1–800/2000 live new born. The alloantibodies are IgG antibodies against the paternal HPA antigens and are responsible for destruction of platelets in the foetus or the newborn. Almost 80% of the instances of FNAIT are a consequence of maternal and foetal incompatibility to HPA-1a, the rest 20% results from incompatibility to HPA-5b on GPIa and other HPAs [57]. In addition to HPA antigens, antibodies against CD36 glycoprotein a member of class B scavenger receptor family [58] is also implicated in the causal of FNAIT. A case study reported, maternal deficiency in expression of CD36 protein lead to maternal immunization against CD36 protein (anti-NAK) [59]. The clinical impact of NAIT is related with maternal immunization against CD36 is analogous to that observed in infants affected by HPA specific antibodies [60].

Alloantibody production by maternal immune system requires the presentation of antigen to maternal T-cell through HLA class II molecules. It was reported that HPA-1a alloimmunization is mediated by interaction of HPA-1a peptides to HLA DRB3*01:01 molecule [57, 61]. This may be a consequence of feto-maternal haemorrhage, which can happen during delivery or abortion, as a consequence of platelet leakage into maternal circulation [62]. Maternal IgG alloantibody thus formed is progressively transported to the foetus through the neonatal Fc receptor, whereas the IgA and IgM are not transported as there are no specific receptors for them. Once through the placenta, the maternal alloantibody opsonises the foetal platelets thereby resulting in their destruction and leading to thrombocytopenia [62–64].

The clinical indication of FNAIT differs from asymptomatic thrombocytopenia to life threatening intracranial haemorrhage (ICH) [57]. Intraparenchymal haemorrhage in the temporal lobe is also most often noticed in FNAIT [65]. Studies have also shown that antibodies against HPA-1a antigen or thrombocytopenia may also result in decreased birth weight and a very low weight for gestational age which presents a health risk later in life [66]. In many of the FNAIT instance, the illness presents as, petechiae, hematomas, haemoptysis, retinal bleeding and haematuria [57, 67]. Occasionally, the bleeding due to FNAIT is diagnosed during foetal life in ultrasound abnormalities [68]. Without routine screening for HPA antibodies the disease is mostly detected after the delivery of the first affected child. Thus, making antenatal treatment and diagnosis possible only for subsequent pregnancies in order to prevent recurrence of severe FNAIT [69]. FNAIT may be diagnosed using antibody detection methods using serological or ELISA based techniques or by platelet typing using PCR-based assays.

The immediate treatment for thrombocytopenia in case of severe bleeding is platelet transfusion [68, 70]. In addition to transfusion intravenous immunoglobulin IVIG can be provided to prolong the survival of incompatible platelets and reduce the overall impact of thrombocytopenia [71, 72]. The most favourable antenatal treatment in order to prevent bleeding complications in pregnancies with FNAIT is non-invasive IVIG treatment on weekly basis [68]. In FNAIT resulting due to anti-CD36 glycoprotein intrauterine transfusions with compatible RBC and CD36 null platelets are useful in preventing the hazardous clinical effect of the disease [73].

4.3 Neonatal alloimmune neutropenia (NAN)

Neonatal alloimmune neutropenia (NAN) is a very rare disorder, but is a life threatening disorder of the neonates. The occurrence of NAN has been estimated to be 1 in 1000/6000 live births. NAN occurs due to maternal sensitization to incompatible paternal foetal granulocyte antigens. The maternal alloantibodies formed against the foetal granulocytes are transported through the placenta which thereby causes the destruction of foetal granulocytes [74].

Maternal alloantibodies against granulocyte-specific antigens HNA-1a and HNA-1b have been accounted widely to cause NAN. Antibodies to Fc gamma RIIb (CD16) and HNA-2a granulocyte antigen are infrequently involved in neonatal neutropenia, if mother is HNA-1 null phenotype [74, 75]. A case study has also reported the involvement of HNA-4b as a causative of severe NAN [76].

Neutropenia in neonates is a self-limiting disorder and lasts for only few weeks, but in some instances, it can prevail for as long as 6 months. In the course of this period, neonates are at severe risk of acquiring infection [75]. Symptomatic neonate suffering NAN frequently present with retarded umbilical cord separation, skin infections, otitis media, or pneumonia within 15 days of life. Most of the infections that occur are mild, but it may at times turn severe. The fatality rate because of NAN has been noted to be around 5%. The severity of NAN is dependent on concentration and the subclass of IgG present [74].

The immune neutropenia correlates with granulocytes specific antibodies present in the serum and can be diagnosed [75] using the granulocyte agglutination test (GAT), the granulocyte immunofluorescence test (GIFT), the monoclonal antibody immobilization of granulocyte antigens assay (MAIGA), an assay called as extracted granulocyte immunofluorescence assay (EGIFA) measures the anti-HNA-1a, -1b, and/or -2 antibodies in the sera. The use of EGIFA assay has been reported to improve the diagnosis and clinical management of patient suspected to have NAN [77]. The treatment for NAN is still a matter of discussion, but the options used for the management of NAN include antibiotics, intravenous immunoglobulin (IVIG), corticosteroids, and human granulocyte colony-stimulating factor (rhG-CSF) [78].

5. Conclusions

Table 1 summarizes the implication of HLA antigens in complications related to pregnancy. Though it is now well identified that the HLA plays major role in pregnancy, placentation and immune modulation to maintain an immune-tolerance

Disease/disorder	Associated HLA allele/ class	Study findings/outcomes	Reference
Rh isoimmunization	HLA A3, B17, CW2 and DR4.	Inheritance of HLA HLA A3, B17, Cw2 and DR4 increased the risk of Rh immunization.	Kumar et al. [79]
NAIT	HLA-DRB3*0101.	Presence of HLA-DRB3*0101 restricted CD4+ cells specific for HPA-1a antigen in alloimmunized women. Implicates strong association of DRB3*0101 in immunization of pregnant women against foetal HPA-1a antigen.	Ahlen et al. [61]

Disease/disorder	Associated HLA allele/class	Study findings/outcomes	Reference
Reduced birth weight of foetus with NAIT	Maternal anti-HLA class I antibodies.	Increased level of maternal anti-HLA class I antibodies in thrombocytopenic neonates are associated with reduce foetal growth.	Dahl et al. [80]
Reproductive failure (recurrent miscarriages and pre-eclampsia)	Group 2 HLA-C alleles (C2).	Foetus expresses both maternally and paternally inherited HLA-C antigens. Substantial increase in the risk for reproductive disorders with mother possessing KIR “AA” genotype and foetus expressing more C2 copies than mother.	Hiby et al. [35]
Recurrent spontaneous abortion	HLA-G with 14 bp polymorphism and SNP 3127(C/G) in the 3′UTR.	Substantial increased frequencies of the genotypes with 14 bp polymorphism and the SNP3127 (C/G) in the 3′UTR in RSA women of Caucasian origin.	Larsen et al. [81]
Recurrent pregnancy loss (RPL)	−1573T > C and −1746C > A SNPs in the promoter of the HLA-G gene HLA-G promoter region haplotype H1(ATCCAGGTAC GCAA) H2(CTTCGAGAAC GCAG).	SNP −1573T > C and −1746C > A in the promoter region of HLA-G gene are associated with RPL H1 is associated with a decreased and H2 is associated with an increased risk of RPL.	Yazdani et al. [29]
Pre-eclampsia	HLA-G with 14 bp polymorphism.	Increased frequencies of the +14 insertion/deletion HLA-G genotype of offspring were associated with severe and early onset of pre-eclampsia in Chinese population.	Zhang et al. [82]
Secondary recurrent miscarriage	HY (male specific minor histocompatibility antigen).	Aberrant maternal immune response against foetal HY antigen play a role in secondary recurrent miscarriage and other pregnancy complications.	Christiansen et al. [40]
Still birth	HY-restricting HLA class II alleles.	Maternal carriage of HY-restricting HLA class II alleles decreases long-term chance of live birth in women with RPL after a boy.	Kolte et al. [41]

Table 1.
Role of HLA in pregnancy disease/disorders.

state. This in turn results in foetus being well accepted by the maternal immune system. Alloimmunization and other pregnancy complications result due to maladapted immune system when the maternal immune system is unable to maintain an immune tolerance state towards the foetus.

Conflict of interest

The authors declare no conflict of interest.

Author details

Meenakshi Singh*, Jyoti Rajak, Shalaka Kadam and Sunil B. Rajadhyaksha
HLA and Immunogenetics Laboratory, Department of Transfusion Medicine, Tata Memorial Hospital, Mumbai, India

*Address all correspondence to: meenakshisingha@gmail.com

References

[1] Medawar PB. Some immunological and endocrinological problems raised by the evolution of viviparity in vertebrates. Symposia of the Society for Experimental Biology. 1953;**44**:320-338

[2] Hunt JS, Langat DK, McIntire RH, Morales PJ. The role of HLA-G in human pregnancy. Reproductive Biology and Endocrinology. 2006;**4**(Suppl 1):S10. DOI: 10.1186/1477-7827-4-S1-S10

[3] Hviid TV. HLA-G in human reproduction: Aspects of genetics, function and pregnancy complications. Human Reproduction Update. 2006;**12**(3):209-232

[4] Peltier MR. Immunology of term and preterm labor. Reproductive Biology and Endocrinology. 2003;**1**:122

[5] Porrett PM. Biologic mechanisms and clinical consequences of pregnancy alloimmunization. American Journal of Transplantation. 2018;**18**:1059-1067

[6] Obeagu EI. Hemolytic disease of the newborn: A review. International Journal of Pharmacotherapy. 2015;**5**(1):XX-XX

[7] Koelewijn JM, Vrijkotte TG, De Haas M, Van Der Schoot CE, Bonsel GJ. Risk factors for the presence of non-rhesus D red blood cell antibodies in pregnancy. BJOG. 2009;**116**:655-664

[8] Hudson LE, Allen RL. Leukocyte Ig-like receptors—A model for MHC class I disease associations. Frontiers in Immunology. 2016;**7**:281

[9] Ober C. HLA and pregnancy: The paradox of the fetal allograft. American Journal of Human Genetics. 1998;**62**:1-5

[10] He X, Xu L, Liu Y, Zeng Y. Identification of a novel HLA-F allele—HLA-F*010102. Tissue Antigens. 2004;**63**:181-183

[11] Allard M, Oger R, Benlalam H, Florenceau L, Echasserieau K, et al. Soluble HLA-I/peptide monomers mediate antigen-specific CD8 T cell activation through passive peptide exchange with cell-bound HLA-I molecules. Journal of Immunology. 2014;**192**(11):5090-5097. DOI: 10.4049/jimmunol.1303226

[12] Leddon SA, Sant AJ. Generation of MHC class II-peptide ligands for CD4 T-cell allorecognition of MHC class II molecules. Current Opinion in Organ Transplantation. 2010;**15**(4):505-511. DOI: 10.1097/MOT.0b013e32833bfc5c

[13] Lee J, Romero R, Xu Y, Kim JS, Park JY, et al. Maternal HLA panel-reactive antibodies in early gestation positively correlate with chronic chorioamnionitis: Evidence in support of the chronic nature of maternal anti-fetal rejection. American Journal of Reproductive Immunology. 2011;**66**(6):510-526

[14] Dahl M, Djurisic S, Hviid TV. The many faces of human leukocyte antigen-G: Relevance to the fate of pregnancy. Journal of Immunology Research. 2014;**2014**:591489

[15] Lynge Nilsson L, Djurisic S, Hviid TV. Controlling the immunological crosstalk during conception and pregnancy: HLA-G in reproduction. Frontiers in Immunology. 2014;**13**(5):198

[16] Hunt JS, Petroff MG, McIntire RH, Ober C. HLA-G and immune tolerance in pregnancy. The FASEB Journal. 2005;**19**(7):681-693

[17] Ellis SA, Sargent IL, Redman CW, McMichael AJ. Evidence for a novel HLA antigen found on human extravillous trophoblast and a choriocarcinoma cell line. Immunology. 1986;**59**:595-601

[18] Morales PJ, Pace JL, Platt JS, Phillips TA, et al. Placental cell expression of HLA-G2 isoforms is limited to the invasive trophoblast phenotype. Journal of Immunology. 2003;**171**:6215-6224

[19] Durmanova V, Homolova M, Drobny J, Shawkatova I, Buc M. Role of HLA-G and other immune mechanisms in pregnancy. Central European Journal of Biology. 2013;**8**:226

[20] Tilburgs T, Evans JH, Crespo ÂC, Strominger JL. The HLA-G cycle provides for both NK tolerance and immunity at the maternal-fetal interface. Proceedings of the National Academy of Sciences of the United States of America. 2015;**112**(43):13312-13317. DOI: 10.1073/pnas.1517724112

[21] Ferreira LMR, Meissner TB, Tilburgs T, Strominger JL. HLA-G: At the interface of maternal-fetal tolerance. Trends in Immunology. 2017;**38**(4):272-286

[22] Sibai B, Dekker G, Kupferminc M. Pre-eclampsia. Lancet. 2005;**365**:785-799. DOI: 10.1016/S0140-6736(05)71003-5

[23] O'Brien M, McCarthy T, Jenkins D, Paul P, Dausset J, Carosella ED, et al. Altered HLA-G transcription in pre-eclampsia is associated with allele specific inheritance: Possible role of the HLA-G gene in susceptibility to the disease. Cellular and Molecular Life Sciences. 2001;**58**(12-13):1943-1949. DOI: 10.1007/PL00000828

[24] Vianna P, Mondadori AG, Bauer ME, Dornfeld D, Chies JA. HLA-G and CD8+ regulatory T cells in the inflammatory environment of pre-eclampsia. Reproduction. 2016;**152**:741-751

[25] Marozio L, Garofalo A, Berchialla P, Tavella AM, et al. Low expression of soluble human leukocyte antigen G in early gestation and subsequent placenta-mediated complications of pregnancy. The Journal of Obstetrics and Gynecology Research. 2017;**43**(9):1391-1396

[26] Rokhafrooz S, Ghadiri A, Ghandil P, Ghafourian M, et al. Association between HLA-G 14 bp gene polymorphism and serum sHLA-G protein concentrations in preeclamptic patients and normal pregnant women. Immunological Investigations. 2018;**47**(6):558-568

[27] Practice Committee of the American Society for Reproductive Medicine. Evaluation and treatment of recurrent pregnancy loss: A committee opinion. Fertility and Sterility. 2012;**98**(5):1103-1111. DOI: 10.1016/j.fertnstert.2012.06.048

[28] Guo W, Fang L, Li B, Xiao X, Chen S, et al. Decreased human leukocyte antigen-g expression by mir-133a contributes to impairment of proinvasion and proangiogenesis functions of decidual nK cells. Frontiers in Immunology. 2017;**8**:741

[29] Yazdani N, Khaniani MS, Bastami M, Ghasemnejad T, et al. HLA-G regulatory variants and haplotypes with susceptibility to recurrent pregnancy loss. International Journal of Immunogenetics. 2018;**45**:181-189

[30] Burton GJ, Woods AW, Jauniaux E, Kingdom JC. Rheological and physiological consequences of conversion of the maternal spiral arteries for utero placental blood flow during human pregnancy. Placenta. 2009;**30**:473-482

[31] Moffett-King A. Natural killer cells and pregnancy. Nature Reviews. Immunology. 2002;**2**:656-663

[32] Brosens I, Pijnenborg R, Vercruysse L, Romero R. The 'great obstetrical syndromes' are associated with disorders of deep placentation.

American Journal of Obstetrics and Gynecology. 2011;**204**:3193-3201. DOI: 10.1016/j.ajog.2010.08.009

[33] Parham P. MHC class I molecules and KIRs in human history, health and survival. Nature Reviews. Immunology. 2005;**5**:201-214. DOI: 10.1038/nri1570

[34] Hiby SE, Regan L, Lo W, Farrell L, et al. Association of maternal killer-cell immunoglobulin-like receptors and parental HLA-C genotypes with recurrent miscarriage. Human Reproduction. 2008;**23**(4):972-976

[35] Hiby SE, Apps R, Sharkey AM, Farrell LE, Gardner L, Mulder A, et al. Maternal activating KIRs protect against human reproductive failure mediated by fetal HLA-C2. The Journal of Clinical Investigation. 2010;**120**:4102-4110

[36] Bari R, Bell T, Leung WH, Vong QP, et al. Significant functional heterogeneity among KIR2DL1 alleles and a pivotal role of arginine 245. Blood. 2009;**114**:5182-5190. DOI: 10.1182/blood-2009-07-231977

[37] Hiby SE, Apps R, Chazara O, Farrell LE, et al. Maternal KIR in combination with paternal HLA-C2 regulate human birth weight. Journal of Immunology. 2014;**192**(11):5069-5073. DOI: 10.4049/jimmunol.1400577

[38] Popli R, Sahaf B, Nakasone H, Lee JY, Miklos DB. Clinical impact of H-Y alloimmunity. Immunologic Research. 2014;**58**(2-3):249-258

[39] Christiansen OB. Reproductive immunology. Molecular Immunology. 2013;**55**(1):8-15

[40] Christiansen OB, Steffensen R, Nielsen HS. Anti-HY responses in pregnancy disorders. American Journal of Reproductive Immunology. 2011;**66**(Suppl 1):93-100

[41] Kolte AM, Steffensen R, Christiansen OB, Nielsen HS. Maternal HY-restricting HLA class II alleles are associated with poor long-term outcome in recurrent pregnancy loss after a boy. American Journal of Reproductive Immunology. 2016;**76**(5):400-405. DOI: 10.1111/aji.12561

[42] Christiansen OB, Kolte AM, Dahl M, Larsen EC, Steffensen R, Nielsen HS, et al. Maternal homozygocity for a 14 base pair insertion in exon 8 of the HLA-G gene and carriage of HLA class II alleles restricting HY immunity predispose to unexplained secondary recurrent miscarriage and low birth weight in children born to these patients. Human Immunology. 2012;**73**:699-705

[43] Fasano RM. Hemolytic disease of the fetus and newborn in the molecular era. Seminars in Fetal & Neonatal Medicine. 2016;**21**:28-34

[44] de Haas M, Finning K, Massey E, Roberts DJ. Anti-D prophylaxis: Past, present and future. Transfusion Medicine (Oxford, England). 2014;**24**:1e7

[45] Costumbrado J, Ghassemzadeh S. Rh incompatibility. In: StatPearls. Treasure Island (FL): StatPearls Publishing; 2018

[46] American College of Obstetricians and Gynecologists. Prevention of Rh D alloimmunization. Practice bulletin No. 181. Obstetrics and Gynecology. 2017;**130**:e57-e70

[47] Moise KJ, Argoti PS. Management and prevention of red cell alloimmunization in pregnancy: A systematic review. Obstetrics and Gynecology. 2012;**120**:1132-1139

[48] Ghesquière L, Garabedian C, Coulon C, Verpillat P, et al. Management of red blood cell alloimmunization in pregnancy. Journal of Gynecology

Obstetrics and Human Reproduction. 2018;**47**(5):197-204

[49] Bowman J. Thirty-five years of Rh prophylaxis. Transfusion. 2003;**43**:1661-1666

[50] Bowman JM. The prevention of Rh immunization. Transfusion Medicine Reviews. 1988;**2**:129-150

[51] Geaghan SM. Diagnostic laboratory technologies for the fetus and neonate with isoimmunization. Seminars in Perinatology. 2011;**35**:148-154

[52] Van Der Schoot CE, Tax GH, Rijnders RJ, De Haas M, Christiaens GC. Prenatal typing of Rh and kell blood group system antigens, the edge of a watershed. Transfusion Medicine Reviews. 2004;**17**(1):31-44

[53] Bowman JM. Hemolytic disease (erythroblastosis fetalis). In: Creasy RK, Resnik R, editors. Maternal-Fetal Medicine. 4th ed. Philadelphia: WB Saunders; 1999. pp. 736-767

[54] Gariod S, Brossard Y, Poissonnier M-H, Vuilliez B, Deutsch V, et al. Kell alloimmunization in pregnancy. Journal de Gynécologie, Obstétrique et Biologie de la Reproduction. 2004;**33**:637-648

[55] de Haas M, Thurik FF, Koelewijn JM, van der Schoot CE. Haemolytic disease of the fetus and newborn. Vox Sanguinis. 2015;**109**(2):99-113

[56] Ree IMC, Smits-Wintjens VEHJ, van der Bom JG, et al. Neonatal management and outcome in alloimmune hemolytic disease. Hematology. 2017;**10**(7):607-616

[57] Brojer E, Husebekk A, Dębska M, Uhrynowska M, Guz K, et al. Fetal/neonatal alloimmune thrombocytopenia: Pathogenesis, diagnostics and prevention. Archivum Immunologiae et Therapiae Experimentalis (Warsz). 2016;**64**(4):279-290

[58] Silverstein RL, Febbraio M. CD36, a scavenger receptor involved in immunity, metabolism, angiogenesis, and behavior. Science Signaling. 2009;**2**(72):1-8

[59] Taketani T, Ito K, Mishima S, Kanai R, et al. Neonatal isoimmune thrombocytopenia caused by type ICD36 deficiency having novel splicing isoforms of the CD36 gene. European Journal of Hematology. 2008;**81**:70-74

[60] Curtis BR, Ali S, Glazier AM, Ebert DD, et al. Isoimmunization against CD36 (glycoprotein IV): Description of four cases of neonatal isoimmune thrombocytopenia and brief review of the literature. Transfusion. 2002;**42**:1173-1179

[61] Ahlen MT, Husebekk A, Killie MK. T-cell responses associated with neonatal alloimmune thrombocytopenia: Isolation of HPA-1a-specific, HLA-DRB3*0101-restricted CD4+ T cells. Blood. 2009;**113**:3838-3844

[62] Kumpel BM, Manoussaka MS. Placental immunology and maternal alloimmune responses. Vox Sanguinis. 2012;**102**:2-12

[63] Kumpel BM. Pregnancy immunology and maternal alloimmune responses. Vox Sanguinis. 2012;**103**:7

[64] Leach JL, Sedmak DD, Osborne JM, Rahill B, Lairmore MD, Anderson CL. Isolation from human placenta of the IgG transporter, FcRn, and localization to the syncytiotrophoblast-implications for maternal-fetal antibody transport. Journal of Immunology. 1996;**157**:3317-3322

[65] Dale ST, Coleman LT. Neonatal alloimmune thrombocytopenia: Antenatal and postnatal imaging

findings in the pediatric brain. American Journal of Neuroradiology. 2002;**23**:1457-1465

[66] Tiller H, Killie MK, Husebekk A, Skogen B, Ni H, Kjeldsen-Kragh J. Platelet antibodies and fetal growth: Maternal antibodies against fetal platelet antigen 1a are strongly associated with reduced birthweight in boys. Acta Obstetricia et Gynecologica Scandinavica. 2012;**91**:79-86

[67] Mueller-Eckhardt C, Kiefel V, Grubert A, Weisheit M, et al. 348 cases of suspected neonatal alloimmune thrombocytopenia. Lancet. 1989;**1**:363-366

[68] Winkelhorst D, Oepkesa D, Lopriorec E. Fetal and neonatal alloimmune thrombocytopenia: Evidence based antenatal and postnatal management strategies. Expert Review of Hematology. 2017;**10**(8):729-737

[69] Kamphuis MM, Tiller H, van den Akker ES, et al. Fetal and neonatal alloimmune thrombocytopenia: Management and outcome of a large international retrospective cohort. Fetal Diagnosis and Therapy. 2017;**41**(4):251-257

[70] Sola-Visner M, Saxonhouse MA, Brown RE. Neonatal thrombocytopenia: What we do and don't know. Early Human Development. 2008;**84**:499-506

[71] Bussel J. Diagnosis and management of the fetus and neonate with alloimmune thrombocytopenia. Journal of Thrombosis and Hemostasis. 2009;**7**(Suppl. 1):253-257

[72] McQuilten ZK, Wood EM, Savoia H, Cole S. A review of pathophysiology and current treatment for neonatal alloimmune thrombocytopenia (NAIT) and introducing the Australian NAIT registry. Australian and New Zealand Journal of Obstetrics and Gynecology. 2011;**51**:191-198

[73] Xu X, Li L, Xia W, Ding H, Chen D, et al. Successful management of a hydropic fetus with severe anemia and thrombocytopenia caused by anti-CD36 antibody. International Journal of Hematology. 2018;**107**:251-256

[74] Tomicic M, Starcevic M, Zach V, Bingulac-Popovic J, Hundric-Haspl Z. A case of neonatal neutropenia due to anti-fc gamma receptor IIIb isoantibodies treated with recombinant human granulocyte colony stimulating factor. Case Reports in Medicine. 2009:717545

[75] Han TH, Chey MJ, Han KS. A case of neonatal alloimmune neutropenia associated with anti-human neutrophil antigen-1a (HNA-1a) antibody. Journal of Korean Medical Science. 2006;**21**:351-354

[76] Curtis BR, Roman AS, Sullivan MJ, Raven CS, Larison J, Weitekamp LA. Two cases of maternal alloimmunization against human neutrophil alloantigen-4b, one causing severe alloimmune neonatal neutropenia. Transfusion. 2016;**56**(1):101-106. DOI: 10.1111/trf.13287

[77] Onodera R, Kurita E, Taniguchi K, Karakawa S, et al. Anti-human neutrophil antigen-1a, -1b, and -2 antibodies in neonates and children with immune neutropenias analyzed by extracted granulocyte antigen immunofluorescence assay. Transfusion. 2017;**57**(11):2586-2594

[78] Agueda S, Rocha G, Ferreira F, Vítor B, Lima M, Guimarães H. Neonatal alloimmune neutropenia: Still a diagnostic and therapeutical challenge. Journal of Pediatric Hematology/Oncology. 2012;**34**(7):497-499

[79] Kumar US, Ghosh K, Gupte SS, Gupte SC, Mohanty D. Role of HLA antigens in Rh (D) alloimmunized pregnant women from Mumbai,

Maharashtra, India. Journal of Biosciences. 2002;**27**:135-114

[80] Dahl J, Husebekk A, Stuge TB, Tiller H, et al. Maternal anti-HLA class I antibodies are associated with reduced birth weight in thrombocytopenic neonates. Journal of Reproductive Immunology. 2016;**113**:27-34

[81] Larsen MH, Hylenius S, Andersen AM, Hviid TV. The 3′-untranslated region of the HLA-G gene in relation to pre-eclampsia: Revisited. Tissue Antigens. 2010;**75**(3):253-261. DOI: 10.1111/j.1399-0039.2009.01435.x

[82] Zhang Z, Li Y, Zhang LL, Jia LT, Yang XQ. Association of 14 bp insertion/deletion polymorphism of the HLA-G gene in father with severe preeclampsia in Chinese. Tissue Antigens. 2012;**80**:158-164. DOI: 10.1111/j.1399-0039.2012.01907.x